The Role of the
Preceptor

A Guide
for Nurse Educators,
Clinicians, and Managers

2nd Edition

Jean Pieri Flynn, EdD, RN, received her bachelor's degree in nursing from the University of Rochester, Rochester, NY, a master of arts degree in inservice education, a master's degree in medical-surgical nursing and education, and a doctor of education degree in research and nursing administration from Teachers College, Columbia University. Dr. Flynn is currently at New York Presbyterian Hospital in the Performance Improvement Department as a Six Sigma organizational improvement leader. She has had extensive experience in staff development, continuing education, and quality improvement, both as an instructor and as a manager at three large metropolitan teaching hospitals in New York City.

Dr. Flynn has been a presenter at numerous national management workshops and research conferences. She is the author of several articles and two books on leadership, medical-surgical nursing, and teaching strategies.

Madonna C. Stack, MA, MPA, RN, received her bachelor's degree from the University of Pennsylvania, a master's degree in medical-surgical nursing and nursing administration, and a master's degree in public administration in the health care administration program at New York University. She has had experience in critical care, staff development, and continuing education as an instructor, clinician, and manager. In addition, she has had extensive experience in executive-level nursing and hospital administration positions in large metropolitan teaching hospitals in New York City. Ms. Stack is currently an independent health care consultant.

Ms. Stack has served in leadership roles in a number of professional organizations, has been a presenter at numerous national conferences, and has authored articles on critical care nursing, nursing administration, and health care, and a textbook on coronary artery bypass surgery.

The Role of the
Preceptor

A Guide
for Nurse Educators,
Clinicians, and Managers

2nd Edition

Editors:

Jean Pieri Flynn, EdD, RN
Madonna C. Stack, MA, MPA, RN

 Springer Publishing Company

Springer Publishing Company, Inc.
11 West 42nd Street
New York, NY 10036

Acquisitions Editor: Ruth Chasek
Production Editor: Sara Yoo
Cover design by Mimi Flow

06 07 08 09 10 / 5 4 3 2 1

Library of Congress Cataloging-in-Publication Data

The role of the preceptor : a guide for nurse educators, clinicians, and managers / [edited by] Jean Pieri Flynn and Madonna C. Stack. — 2nd ed.
    p. ; cm.
    Includes bibliographical references and index.
    Summary: "This book contains two new chapters on preceptorship in home care settings and distance learning programs. It exemplifies the second edition of this how-to-guide for nursing faculty and clinicians. Flynn and Stack provide a useful and easy-to-follow framework for not only developing and implementing preceptor programs, but also for learning how to precept students and facilitate the development of nursing expertise in both preceptors and preceptees. This second edition includes information on precepting, mentoring, and teaching; a model preceptor program, which includes charts, tables; and a special section on internships, residencies, and mentoring in the nursing program. Overall, the concept of how preceptorship aids in nursing education is shown throughout this book" - Provided by the Publisher.
    ISBN 0-8261-3715-6 (softcover)
    1. Nursing—Study and teaching (Preceptorship)
    [DNLM: 1. Preceptorship—organization & administration. 2. Education, Nursing— organization & administration.   WY 18.5 R744 2006]   I. Flynn, Jean Pieri. II. Stack, Madonna C.

RT74.7.R65 2006
610.73'071'55—dc22   2005013854

Printed in the United States of America by Sheridan Books, Inc.

Contents

Contributors

Barbara Stevens Barnum, PhD, RN, FAAN, a former editor of both *Nursing Leadership Forum* and *Nursing & Healthcare*, is presently a writer and consultant. She previously served in positions at both Columbia University programs of nursing (Medical Center and Teachers College), including holding the directorship, and Division of Health Services, Sciences, and Education at Teachers College, where she also held the Stewart Chair and Chairmanship in the Department of Nursing Education. Dr. Barnum has written widely in areas of nursing management, theory, education, and aspects of spirituality/holistic nursing. Her books include *Nursing Theory: Analysis, Application, Evaluation* (5th ed.); *New Spirituality in Nursing: From Traditional to New Age* (2nd ed.); *The Nurse as Executive* (4th ed., with K. Kerfoot); *Writing for Publication: A Primer for Nurses*; and *The New Healers: Minds and Hands in Complementary Medicine*.

Anne E. Belcher, PhD, RN, AOCN, FAAN, is Senior Associate Dean for Academic Affairs at Johns Hopkins University School of Nursing. She has more than 35 years of experience in nursing education, having taught at the baccalaureate, masters, and doctoral levels. She has held numerous academic administrative positions, including Director of the Undergraduate Program at Thomas Jefferson University, Philadelphia, PA, just prior to joining the faculty at Johns Hopkins. Dr. Belcher's area of expertise is oncology nursing and her research interest is psychosocial aspects of cancer, with a focus on spiritual care. Dr. Belcher holds a bachelor of science in nursing from the University of North Carolina, a master of nursing degree from the University of Washington, Seattle, and a doctorate from the Florida State University, Tallahassee. She is an Advanced Oncology Certified Nurse and a Fellow in the American Academy of Nursing.

Linda R. Conover EdD, MS, RN, received a BSN from St. Anselm College, Manchester, NH, an MS in Community Health

Nursing from Boston University, and an EdD in Higher Education Administration from Vanderbilt University. She is the Director of Distance Nursing Education Programs (RN-BSN, RN-MSN, and MSN) at Saint Joseph's College of Maine in Standish, Maine. Her areas of teaching and expertise are Community Health and Population Focused Practice Nursing, curriculum, and teaching. She consults widely in areas related to nursing education.

Marilyn Hecker, MA, MS, RN, received a bachelor's degree in nursing from Adelphi University, a master's degree in education from Teachers College, Columbia University, and a master's degree in nursing administration from Adelphi University. She is currently Vice President of staff development at Metropolitan Jewish Health System in Brooklyn, New York. Ms. Hecker has worked in home care for many years on Long Island, and in New York City as a clinician and educator, and has successfully implemented a preceptorship program in her current position.

Janet Mackin, EdD, RN, is currently the Dean of both Long Island College Hospital School of Nursing and Phillips Beth Israel School of Nursing in New York City. Dr. Mackin has had a wide variety of educational experiences as a staff development instructor, director of nursing education, and executive director of training. She earned her doctoral degree in the AEGIS Program at Teachers College, Columbia University.

Susan Wiley Nesbitt, MA, MPA, PhD, is the Vice President for the Division of Graduate and Professional Studies at Saint Joseph's College in Maine. She received both her MPA and PhD from the Robert Wagner Graduate School of Public Service at New York University. Her recent publications are in the field of Adult and Distance Education and Learning. She has also published in the area of Health Care Finance.

Ann M. O'Mara, PhD, RN, received her bachelor's degree in nursing from the State University of New York at Buffalo, her master's degree in nursing from Catholic University, Washington, DC, and her doctorate in adult and higher education from the University of Maryland, College Park. Dr. O'Mara is currently Program Director at the National Cancer Institute, National Institutes of Health, and manages the portfolio of investigator-initiated research in the areas of symptom management, and palliative and end-of-life care. Prior to this position, she was on the faculty of the University of Maryland School of Nursing where she coordinated the clinical practicum for senior undergraduate students. Her publications have been in the areas of rewarding staff nurse preceptors, designing and evaluating clinical learning experiences in hospice and end-of-life care, and oncology nursing.

Carmen D. Schmidt, MSN, RN, is Director of Nursing Education and Research for Beth Israel Medical Center and St. Luke's-Roosevelt Hospital in New York City. Ms. Schmidt is responsible for nursing education, orientation, preceptor training programs, and housewide in-service programs. She holds an MSN in Medical Surgical Nursing from Adelphi University.

Deborah Wright Shpritz, PhD, RN, received her diploma in nursing from the Maryland General Hospital School of Nursing, Baltimore, her bachelor's degree in nursing and master's degree in nursing education from the University of Maryland, School of Nursing, Baltimore, and her doctorate in Curriculum Theory and Development from the University of Maryland, College Park. She has more than 20 years experience in academia, working with both undergraduate and graduate students in precepted and nonprecepted courses. Currently she is Program Director for Palliative Care Education at the University of Maryland, School of Medicine, where she coordinates the junior medical student rotation in Hospice and Palliative Care and has developed an online course in End-of-Life Care for medical residents. She is also Adjunct Faculty at the Johns Hopkins School of Nursing. Her recent publications are in the area of education, palliative care, and neuroscience nursing.

Foreword

Excellent preceptorships are essential for contemporary nursing education. There can be no role of greater importance than that of the preceptor, who can shepherd the new entry level or advanced practice nurse as he or she learns an essential new component of the professional role. In the past, the usual model for clinical education at the undergraduate level was for full-time faculty to join their students in clinical settings in order to demonstrate competencies and provide continuous feedback. Today, preceptors join the educational enterprise in many forms. They may be expert nurses in a clinical setting or nurses who, for a variety of reasons, are working part-time and choose to continue a preceptor role as adjunct or part-time clinical faculty. For all preceptors, excellent skills in communication, team building, evaluative skills, and clinical proficiency are key for successful preceptorships. Further, the quality of the clinical agency is central to a positive outcome. It seems self-evident that a student being educated in a clinical setting where patient care outcomes are of the highest quality will learn to practice with the utmost care and the highest expectations for quality nursing.

This book examines and highlights the role of the preceptor and is an important text for every nurse educator, clinician or manager who works with, recruits, or aspires to become a preceptor. The book will be a valuable guide for students as well, as they consider their goals and partner with faculty in the preceptor selection and evaluation process. This book attends to extremely important issues surrounding the preceptor role such as cultural diversity and cultural competency, which are key variables in today's pluralistic society. Differences in preceptor roles and required competencies depending on the clinical setting are also explored. Students deserve highly qualified, competent role models. This text explains the benefits of having the right preceptor at the right time. How a nurse can continue to expect precepting in the employment setting is discussed, with special attention to those newly hired. This text reminds us how each of us has a role to play in ensuring that the preceptor role is all that it can and should be for our profession.

TERRY FULMER, PhD, RN, FAAN
Steinhardt School of Education,
The Erline Perkins McGriff Professor &
Head, Division of Nursing,
New York University

Preface

The idea for the first edition of this book was generated at a colloquium for nurse educators and nurse clinicians. One of the nurse practitioners attending this colloquium said that she liked having students to precept in the clinical setting, but that she had no idea how to plan experiences for these students or how to teach them. This practitioner felt very competent about her knowledge base and about taking care of patients, but she felt inadequate in providing a meaningful clinical experience for students. Although she found several articles about various aspects of precepting in nursing journals, she could locate no book that covered all the essential information. Hence, the first edition was written as a practical "how-to" guide for nursing faculty and for nursing clinicians who were responsible for setting up preceptor programs.

Since the first edition was written 7 years ago, preceptor programs through out the country have grown in numbers, effectiveness and setting. The need for this text, therefore, is even more crucial than at the time of the original edition.

Like the first edition of this book, this text is a practical "how-to" guide for nursing faculty, clinicians and managers. Chapters 1, 2, 3, 4, and 7 have been updated and improved with the addition of new material. Chapter 5, which presents a preceptor model for the home care setting, and chapter 6, which discusses a preceptor model as part of a distance learning program, are both new.

Effective preceptor programs do not happen automatically; they involve careful planning on the part of both preceptor and program administrator. The hope is that this book continues to provide a useful framework for developing and implementing preceptor programs for precepting others; and for facilitating the development of nursing expertise in preceptees in all practice settings. We hope that the present version of the book will prove useful to all members of the nursing profession.

Jean Pieri Flynn
Madonna C. Stack
Editors

Acknowledgments

I want to thank my former students and colleagues in both the acute care and home care settings who have helped me to develop my views and expertise on the preceptor role. I appreciate greatly the assistance, high standards and availability of Ruth Chasek throughout the editing process.

To George Flynn, my husband, I again extend my loving thanks for his patience, support, and active participation in the preparation of this book. Finally, I thank each of the authors who were hardworking and timely in submission of manuscripts, and who provided the expertise so necessary for a book of this nature.

J.P.F.

I want to thank those in the early development of my career who were my preceptors and mentors. Without their guidance, support, and belief in my abilities, I would not have had the career that I have had.

I would also like to thank my friend and colleague, Jean Flynn, for giving me the opportunity to work with her once again. It has been a pleasure.

M.C.S.

CHAPTER 1

Precepting, not Mentoring or Teaching: *Vive la Différence*

Barbara Stevens Barnum

Precepting, of course, is what one defines it to be. In the definition used here, it is different from either teaching or mentoring. What the three share is that they are all based on an essential inequality where one person (teacher, preceptor, mentor) has something to teach that the other, more junior person wants to learn. Although rooted in unequal power, all parties to these relationships may achieve personal and/or professional gains through them.

In order to create generic terms that can be used for all three cases, the senior member in the relationship will be called a *tutor* and the junior member a *pupil*. Although these are rather stuffy terms, they allow us to reserve the more common terms for the subsets. *Instructing* will be used generically. Obviously, the use of these terms in this way is simply a convention for the purposes of this chapter.

Teaching, precepting, and mentoring will be three subsets in the instructing relationship, with precepting falling somewhere between teaching and mentoring on the continuum.

Teaching is a relationship in which someone (the teacher) conveys knowledge (about something) to an individual or group of learners (the students). The relationship is primarily one way, from teacher to student. Even where students are assigned responsibility for presenting information (e.g., symposia or group reports), the teacher still is the arbiter of the information's accuracy and adequacy. Typically, today's teaching is conveyed in directive conversational exchanges, but the traditional lecture is still a common form.

In formal courses, evaluations may take the form of class presentations, tests, papers, or projects receiving feedback. In laboratory courses, there may be individual correction and feedback on experiments, procedures, and various applications. Good teaching probably has more two-way interaction than poor teaching.

Everyone, of course, has had teachers who could hold classes spellbound without students ever saying a word. Most people have had at least one teacher whom they resented because the students were given an inordinate amount of responsibility for conducting the course, with the teacher adding few additional thoughts or clarifications.

Nor does all teaching take place in the formal setting; it can be on-the-spot and incidental. Head nurses teach staff members every day; staff nurses teach their peers. The impetus in both formal and informal situations is that the junior person or persons need to learn something.

In the emotive structure of teaching there is little requirement for an intimate or close relationship between the parties. A teacher may be distant to the students or more friendly with some than with others. Some teachers become motherly, sisterly, or treat students like buddies, but none of these stances is a requirement for effective teaching.

Teaching is about learning *something*, and it is structured around what is to be taught or learned, that is, the content. The personal aspects are secondary.

Mentoring goes to the other extreme of the spectrum. Unlike teaching, which may occur one-to-one or one-to-many, mentoring always takes place in a one-to-one relationship. Here a senior person and a more junior person voluntarily enter a relationship whereby the senior both instructs and, more or less, guides the junior's career and career choices over a sustained period of time— often a lifetime.

What gets conveyed in a mentorship cannot be defined in anyone's curriculum. The content addressed changes as the relationship grows and the people change. Essentially, the mentor instructs in or facilitates whatever the junior person needs to learn (in order to get ahead) at any given time. This may involve knowledge, know-how, politics, philosophic stances, introductions to the right people, or finagled invitations to make important presentations. Name it, and it may enter the mentoring relationship at some stage. As Vance (2002) states, "The leader-mentor plays an essential development role in the professional socialization and the personal and career development of colleagues" (p. 84).

A mentorship may even involve nonprofessional lessons, such as how to promote a career while retaining a spouse, or where to find the best tax accountant. In a mentorship, the personal and the professional are beautifully and messily compounded and intermixed.

Mentorships are never the result of an assignment, although they may grow out of a preceptorship or a teaching relationship. They often occur simultaneously, on the basis of some personal spark, when a work situation brings two people together in a superior–subordinate relationship.

Mentoring is the term nurses prefer when fostering the careers of protégés, partly because most dislike using any terms that are characteristic of the "old boys' " network. Mentoring provides a good two-way interpersonal relationship, in which both parties benefit, though, one could argue, the protégé usually *benefits* more and the mentor usually *invests* more.

The main problem with mentoring is that it lacks equivalent terms like tutor/pupil or teacher/student. This chapter uses mentor/protégé, the latter instead of the more awkward term, *mentee*. The term *protégé* carries some of the right-feeling tone for a mentorship. A mentor is personally invested in the success of the protégé. Indeed, the protégé's success is a measure of the mentor's own success. The term *protégé* connotes that sense of advocacy.

In essence a mentorship is more about the person than about what is taught. The shift is from content to person, from specifics to career development. The emotive structure is important, and the relationship is intimate. Nursing is fortunate in that Sigma Theta Tau International has established the Chiron Mentor-Fellow Program to sponsor selected relationships in this classification.

Precepting, in this definition, falls in between teaching and mentoring. Like mentoring, it is a one-to-one relationship. Even if a person precepts more than one student, each relationship tends to be handled in a one-to-one manner. A preceptorship also is sustained over time, but usually a much shorter time than a mentorship: not a lifetime, perhaps a school term, perhaps a year.

Although mentorships are formed when something clicks between two people, each of whom has something to bring to the other, preceptorships tend to be contractual or informally arranged. Often they occur between people who do not know each other beforehand. Sometimes there is an interview first, if the relationship is to be on the sustained side or if the senior person is considering a number of candidates. Sometimes precepting is an assigned duty, as when an organization assigns someone to orient another to a job or role.

The goals of a preceptorship tend to be definite, even when they are broad in context. For example, an experienced head nurse may precept a new head nurse during the experience of learning to run a unit. True, that's a broad goal, but when the purpose and objectives are deemed to be achieved, the preceptorship ends. Nobody precepts someone else through a lifetime.

Although it resembles the mentorship in being a one-to-one relationship, preceptorship is more like teaching in respect to content. There are learning goals to be achieved and they are professional, not personal.

Yes, preceptorship has a touch of the personal because the evaluation and correction tend to be adjusted on an individual basis. In essence, it is more personal than most teaching, less personal than most mentorships. A preceptorship is more about specific content than a mentorship, but usually about broader, less restrictive content than teaching.

The most difficult thing about a preceptorship is finding an adequate vocabulary to describe it. Teacher/student and mentor/protégé work fine, but preceptor/preceptee? The latter term is too stiff, too derived. For purposes of this chapter, the person who is precepted is labeled an *apprentice*. This term actually fits the relationship quite well. In any domain, an apprentice is there to learn from a master. The experience of the latter and the inexperience of the former set the type of relationship they will have.

The chief characteristics of teaching, precepting, and mentoring are summarized in Table 1.1.

TABLE 1.1 Overview of Teaching, Precepting, and Mentoring

Characteristics	Teaching	Precepting	Mentoring
1. Focus	Content to be taught	Experiential objectives to be achieved	Whatever junior person needs to learn to function in the envisioned role. Focus is on the best way for a protégé to achieve
2. Goals	Professional in nature; not individualized to the learner	Professional in nature; clearly defined	Professional or personal; defined over time
3. Learning Context	Classes/conferences	Workplace/performance in the practice setting	Workplace/with informal, on-the-spot education/feedback
4. Relationship	One-to-many/One-to-one; usually contractual; ends when content delivered	One-to-one; contractual; time limits set at the start	One-to-one; relationship sustained over indefinite period of time
5. Content	Rules, norms, principles, generalizations	Subtleties and varieties in real-world applications	Adapting one's own style and talents to real-world applications
6. Student	Identified as learner	Identified as experienced learner	May be identified as skilled learner or as subordinate
7. Evaluation	By tests, papers, projects, presentations	Assessment of individual performance; may include projects	Retroactive analysis of individual performance
8. Reimbursement	Teacher paid, tuitions/fees	Varies from payment to volunteer post	Seldom involves exchange of monies

LEARNING CONTEXT

Now that the three basic instructing/learning relationships have been differentiated, the contexts in which they occur must be examined, chiefly because the context determines what learning methods will be used. Teaching tends to be the stuff of which classes, demonstration laboratories, and conferences are made. Mentoring, on the other hand, is more closely involved with informal, on-the-spot education based exclusively on assessment of the protégé's performance on the problem of the moment.

Again, precepting falls in the middle. Some learning situations in a preceptorship may resemble teaching. For example, the apprentice may be given reading assignments, projects, and other materials with which to interact. Often the progress of the apprentice will be judged on these matters as well as on performance. Nevertheless, of the three forms of instruction, precepting tends to be the one most exclusively related to actual practice performance in a given role.

REIMBURSEMENT

One of the simplest and most pragmatic ways to differentiate among our three tutor/pupil relationships is by looking at the flow of cold hard cash. Simply put, for sustained or formal relationships, teachers expect to get paid, whether they are faculty or staff development instructors. For incidental teaching, the "payment" may be producing a coworker who no longer asks so many questions. Or, for patient teaching, the payment may be the rewarding sense that the patient will manage when he/she gets home.

There is not enough money in the world, however, to reimburse a mentor. These are voluntary relationships given out of the goodness of the mentor's heart. Mentorships are never formal agreements. If they are, they are actually preceptorships. If reimbursement takes place, it may be in the form of personal gifts now and then. The mentor usually is on the giving end more often here, too. After all, the protégé is likely to be of an age to have weddings, childbirths, and new positions to celebrate. What does the mentor have? Perhaps a retirement if she lives long enough. Mentor rewards exist, of course, but they tend to consist in pride in one's accomplishments with the protégé.

Once again, preceptorships fall somewhere in between. Some nurses volunteer to be preceptors "out of the kindness of their hearts," but it is a professional kindness rather than a kindness to a particular apprentice. In some organizations preceptors gain status, and in some places salaries are adjusted to compensate for the added responsibility.

Payment may be influenced by the programs from which the apprentice comes and the site of the preceptorship. Apprentices may come from the same institution as the preceptors. For example an experienced head nurse may precept a new head nurse. Intrainstitutional preceptors are seldom paid.

Alternately, apprentices may come from different institutions. For example collegiate nursing students may seek preceptorships in care delivery institutions. In these interinstitutional arrangements, the care delivery institution typically receives some reimbursement for providing preceptors. Some institutions continue to precept students "for the sake of the coming generation of nurses." This generosity, alas, is fading as institutions find themselves under the financial pressures of managed care. Precepting, like other forms of instruction, takes a lot of valuable time, and time is money. Where nursing departments are held accountable for producing income, they are likely to set fees for preceptorships.

GENERALIZATIONS AND INSTANTIATIONS

Another difference among the forms of instruction is that teaching almost always deals with presenting rules, norms, principles, and generalities, whereas the other forms more commonly cope with exceptions to the rule. In teaching/learning, for example, one learns the norms of anemia, not *how differently the symptoms may appear* from one patient to the next. Teaching is the task of conveying the universals.

Of course, some things really are universal; for example, one should always clear the airway before administering resuscitation. But many so-called universals are more tricky. Establishing rapport with a patient may be a good dictate—in most situations—but how one does this will differ radically from one patient to the next and from one nurse to the next. Rotating weekends equally among staff may be a good principle for any head nurse, but it may not work if one of her staff is in school Mondays and Wednesdays, another is a Seventh Day Adventist, and one party lover considers Friday and Saturday to be the weekend.

Here is where preceptorships and mentorships have a great advantage. If teaching gives the universals, these other forms of education build an appreciation in the learner of the subtleties and varieties (instantiations) that exist in the real world. That is where these forms of education take place: in the workplace, not in the classroom (unless one is orienting a student teacher).

ROLE MODELING

The notion of role modeling brings up another major difference in teaching methods. Precepting and mentoring involve a lot of role modeling followed by moments of one-to-one reflection on the mentor's/preceptor's performance. Mentoring and precepting may also involve opportunities for the protégé/apprentice to perform under the watchful eye of the senior person, again followed by retrospective analysis or on-the-spot correction if possible.

Often in role taking and role modeling, there is a subtle difference between precepting and mentoring. In precepting, the apprentice is known as, and identified as, a learner. In mentoring, that may or may not be the case. For example, a vice president for nursing may serve as a mentor for an assistant vice president who is not in a student role but in a subordinate role. Here the junior person is an informal learner picking up skills, responsibilities, or strategies in preparation for an eventual upward movement. Meanwhile the protégé holds full job accountability in the institution. The apprentice is rarely a permanent staff person in this sense. Some nurse internships follow a preceptor model, however; but these interns seldom have full job accountability until they complete the internship.

NURSING TRADITIONS

For generations *teaching* was the dominant technique in the education of nurses. Indeed, nurses went out of their way to avoid the notion of apprenticeship. Learning on the job (as it was envisioned in an earlier era) was low class and nonacademic. It has taken generations to recognize the mistake in nursing's overreacting against the apprenticeship model. Indeed, Benner's work (Benner, 1984, 2000; Benner, Tanner, & Chesla, 1996) brought home the fact that not everything gets learned in a classroom or in one return demonstration.

In a complex and dynamic field like nursing, the instantiations may not look much like the schoolroom generalizations at all. In nursing, patients, employees, and bosses don't act like averages, and all the generalizations learned in classrooms may not apply to Patient X in situation Y. One may go for months or years before meeting the patient with a "normal" heart attack or an "average" case of diabetes.

Indeed, to find a textbook case of anything is quite astounding. This is why a student who can recite the definition of classic denial may miss identifying such a syndrome in her patient. Benner's expert nurse is one who has been around the institutions long enough to develop a certain savvy. The expert is accustomed to patients and situations that don't resemble the textbook. She can diagnose and respond to the atypical, recognizing an instantiation. That is why Benner's nurse is not likely to say, "This is a case of denial." She is more likely to say, "Mr. X reminds me of a patient I had last year. He was clever at hiding his denial too."

There are some things that can only be learned by a great deal of experience with a lot of instantiations: hence the need for apprenticeships. Precepting, then, deals with a level of reality that cannot be adequately conveyed in the typical teaching model.

ROLE INCULCATION

Sometimes, a big part of mentorships and preceptorships is giving the protégé/apprentice a chance to *be* the role, to internalize the role. Just like new grandmothers often protest that they don't "feel" like grandmothers, graduation does not make a nurse feel like a nurse, and promotion does not make a staff nurse feel like a head nurse. New roles, like new robes, have to be worn awhile before they fit comfortably.

Teaching is not designed to foster role inculcation, but preceptorships and mentorships can achieve this. That is why people say roles are not taught, but caught.

WHICH MODEL? WHEN AND WHERE?

This is not to say that precepting and mentoring are better than teaching: they are just different. Each form of instructing has its place, and usually one cannot be substituted for the other with much efficiency. Teaching usually comes first. After all, one cannot learn the exceptions unless one knows the rules. For most types of learning, teaching is more efficient than trial-and-error apprenticeship in the workplace. So most faculty members, for example, teach a bit about the brain and its potential deficits before turning students loose on a neurological ward.

What formal teaching cannot do is inculcate a role or provide diverse experience. Nor do teachers provide role models apart from "teacher" models. A teacher functioning as a teacher does *not* model staff nurse behavior: she models teacher behavior. Maybe that is why so many new graduates want to be teachers. That is what they have seen if they were "protected" from becoming close to practicing nurses during their learning experiences.

A role model is someone already doing the job to which the learner aspires, or doing the same job as the learner but doing it more effectively. Here the form of instruction we need is work experience or assisted experience in the form of a preceptorship or mentorship.

Teaching is a cost-effective form of instruction. One can lecture to a group of hundreds as easily as to a group of two. Even the feedback can be mass managed with objective tests. But one-to-one relationships give a sort of feedback and correction that simply is not available any other way.

Still, we see some subtle differences between the preceptorship and the mentorship. The good preceptor may focus on having the apprentice "do it right," in other words, focus on skill acquisition. A skilled mentor, however, is able to ask, What is the best way for this particular protégé, replete with flaws, faults, talents, and opportunities, to achieve?

A WORD ABOUT METHODS

Each form of instruction has methods of conveying information that work, those that work less efficiently, and those that don't work at all. Some of the worst errors in instruction occur when the tutor selects methods that best fit with other systems.

Let us look first at formal teaching, particularly classroom teaching. Here the instructor has a wealth of appropriate methods:

lecture, provided it adds insight into what the students can learn from reading their assignments; case studies that focus on the "average patient or condition"; directed discussions, provided they are really directed; demonstrations of procedures and practices; and other classical methods. The fancy ones include symposium, debate, case presentation, and problem studies, among others.

Although we tend to value classroom teaching more than other methods, the truth is that it is one of the easiest forms of instruction. Any teacher with just a bit of cleverness will soon figure out which classroom methods work best.

Informal teaching is a bit more challenging. Take, for example, the nurse who tries to teach insulin administration and the basics of diabetes care to a newly diagnosed patient. Here the subject matter becomes difficult to convey because a lot of emotional things get in the way. First, the patient may not have truly accepted the diagnosis yet—even if he thinks he has. The patient who cannot quite believe he is a diabetic is working against himself when he tries to "learn" diabetic care.

Additionally, if the patient happens to be ill, the situation adds to the stress. Learning that one is diabetic is stress enough, but if the diabetes is discovered in the wake of a serious imbalance or as part of a surgical workup for another condition, the stress is doubled. All the literature on teaching tells us that people are very inefficient learners when under stress. Yet, ironically, much of our teaching takes place in the hospital or other health care setting when the patient/learner is under great stress.

The teacher, in this case, must assume that the task will take teaching, reteaching, and lots of corrective feedback. Audio-visuals will be most useful here, as will take-home materials that can be reviewed when the patient is under less stress. The same stress factors, of course, will pertain to a nervous nurse being taught to do peritoneal dialysis or any procedure she perceives as complex.

Mentoring may require a bit of teaching, but mostly it involves retroactive analysis of the protégé's performance in some situation or on some task. Proactive preparation for the given task may also be needed. Usually the tasks involved here are more complex than nursing procedures. For example, the protégé and mentor might do a retrospective analysis of how the protégé performed in running a meeting. They would look at what worked, what did not, and what should be tried the next time. Mentoring sometimes involves bailing out a protégé who gets in over his/her head.

Mentoring also may include discussing the mentor's performance on some task, again with proactive or retrospective review. This is the role-modeling aspect. An insightful mentor does not expect the protégé to become a duplicate copy, but allows room for differences in style and different capabilities.

Another important part of mentoring is promoting the protégé's career. This is done in numerous ways, from recommending the protégé for progressively more important positions, to opening doors to important people, to helping the protégé solve career-impeding problems.

Just as we do not consider it very good mothering when the 35-year-old single son still lives with his mother, we do not consider it good mentoring when the protégé is kept in eternal servitude, never allowed to fly solo. There are many cases when a protégé has been kept in thrall for too long—for example, someone who has been an assistant to her mentor for 20 years. This is a failed relationship that serves the mentor all too well and stunts the protégé's growth. The ideal is somewhere between *All About Eve* and indentured servitude.

Precepting goes wrong when an insecure preceptor tries to convert the experience into teaching. In this case, the preceptor teaches the apprentice procedures, gives reading assignments and little teaching sessions, but never lets the apprentice get his/her hands dirty in the real world, where the precepted role takes place. Too much "mothering" or too much protection from the clinical arena (often by withdrawal into conferences) are the errors on one side. Application of the sink-or-swim principle is an error in the opposite direction.

STUDENT CLINICAL EXPERIENCE: A SPECIAL CASE

Student clinical experience is a unique form of learning. Although it is less valued (by the institution) than classroom teaching or research, the truth is that it is equally or more difficult to do effectively. A good clinical teacher should be praised and covered with honors.

Good clinical instruction is a blend of teaching and precepting. The teaching part is easy. Indeed, the new and inexpert clinical teacher is the one who focuses on finding "procedures" for the students to do—the most normative part of the clinical role. In addition to this, the insecure teacher withdraws students from the clinical area at the slightest excuse. Why? Because she is comfortable *teaching*—and the clinical conference comes closest to that method.

In contrast, the good clinical preceptor immerses the students in the clinical environment and challenges them to see the irregularities and differences between patients and staff alike. This instructor helps each student consider options when the first one fails. In this respect, instruction must be individualized. After all, each student is different and each faces a different clinical assignment.

What are the chief ingredients to be found in clinical instruction? There are at least three major responsibilities beyond teaching tasks. First, the instructor must spark the student's intellectual curiosity. "Mr. Smith is a lovely shade of brown, but did you notice, according to the chart, that he's Irish? Doesn't that strike you as curious?"

The next task is to teach the student to recognize inconsistencies. That is done by presenting problems or things that do not seem quite right. "Your patient, Mr. Jones, is the funniest, most outgoing guy I've ever seen. Here he is, going for a second major surgery in the morning, and he's joking and laughing with everyone. Most patients would be anxious or scared. What do you think is going on with Mr. Jones?"

The last task is accurate labeling of patients who are not typical with appropriate normative labels. One might call this accurate interpretation. The student who knows the definition of passive aggression may mistake it for dependency in Mrs. Doe until she builds a bit of experience. The good preceptor will help her make a better fit of labels to patients.

These clinical skills (labeling, seeing inconsistencies, and having an insatiable curiosity) may or may not be discrete items, but they all have something to do with forests and trees. The forest is the principle, the ruling norm; the trees are the instantiations found in patients.

Not every effective tutor will draw rigid boundaries around instruction according to form. However, being aware of the differences among teaching, precepting, and mentoring may help the instructor make a wiser choice in how to convey information.

SUMMARY

There are at least three basic points on the instruction continuum: teaching, precepting, and mentoring. Each instructional strategy has its own virtues and its own limitations. Together, they uniquely complement each other. Their differences provide different perspectives as well as serve different goals.

Teaching is content focused; mentoring is student focused. Precepting, like teaching, is content focused, albeit the content tends to be broader, but at the same time it is like mentoring in that it also is student focused. Here again, precepting resembles teaching in that the student is taught and evaluated on specific, predetermined objectives.

Experiences of all three sorts of instruction enhance the learning and the career of a nurse. All of these tutor–pupil relationships serve to speed up the learning that occurs by simple immersion in the phenomena (otherwise known as trial and error learning, or working for a living).

REFERENCES

Benner, P. (1984). *From novice to expert: Excellence and power in clinical nursing practice*. Menlo Park, CA: Addison-Wesley.

Benner, P. (2000). *From novice to expert: Excellence and power in clinical nursing practice* (Commemorative Edition). Menlo Park, CA: Addison-Wesley.

Benner, P., Tanner, C. A., & Chesla, C. A. (1996). *Expertise in nursing practice: Caring, clinical judgment, and ethics*. New York: Springer Publishing.

Vance, C. (2002, Winter). Leader as mentor. *Nursing Leadership Forum*, 7(2), 83–90.

CHAPTER 2

Adult Learning Concepts

Susan Wiley Nesbitt

Research and publications related to adult education have increased significantly in the last 20 years (Brookfield, 1986; Knowles, Holton, & Swanson, 1998; Merriam, 2001; Merriam & Brockett, 1997; Mezirow & Associates, 2000). This body of knowledge provides helpful guidelines to educators working with adults. The writings from two different groups of researchers are especially relevant for preceptors. The first group that includes the writings of Malcolm Knowles, Edward F. Horton, and Richard A. Swanson focuses on the concept of andragogy. The basis of this concept is a set of assumptions about adults which, when considered in the process of educating adults, will shape and focus that education so it is meaningful and appropriate for them. The second, Jack Mezirow, focuses on transformational learning. The nucleus of this concept is that people do not acquire new knowledge by memorizing facts. Instead they acquire new knowledge by integrating new information with previously held ideas, values, etc., thus "transforming" their knowledge. In a preceptorship a person, known as the preceptor, with selected knowledge or experience guides an apprentice as he or she acquires similar knowledge or experience. Thus, using the assumptions on which andragogy is based and understanding that the apprentice should build this new knowledge on information they already possess will assist the preceptor to develop a meaningful experience for the apprentice. This chapter begins with a brief overview of both andragogy and transformational learning. Based on these works, eight useful guidelines for the development of effective preceptor experiences are examined.

ANDRAGOGY:
THE ART AND SCIENCE OF TEACHING ADULTS

Although the term *andragogy* was developed in the 1800s, it became well-known through the work of Knowles. Andragogy assumes that "adults are self-directed, have abundant resources within themselves for learning, want to develop their skills in their social roles, and want to apply their learning immediately" (Hancock, 2003, p. 15; Knowles et al., 1998). Knowles views learning as occurring on a continuum from a teacher-centered approach or pedagogy, which is the art and science of teaching children, to a learner-centered approach or andragogy, which is the art and science of teaching adults.

Six assumptions form the basis for andragogy. They are:

1. The motivation to learn increases for adults when they either have a specific need for the knowledge such as when they are working toward a job promotion or when they have a specific interest in a topic.

2. A person's stage of life will impact what they are motivated to learn. For example, people seeking to improve their basic clinical skills will not be interested in the managerial skills needed by a Nurse Manager. However, after they have worked several years as a nurse they could be very interested in being promoted to a managerial position. Now they would be interested in a leadership course.

3. It is said that we remember only 5% from a lecture and more than 90% with applied learning. Thus, when adults can learn through experience their motivation to learn will be greater and their retention of the knowledge better.

4. While adult learning needs to be structured so no important concepts are missed, it is important to understand that adults want to be self-directed. Once a person accepts responsibility for himself it is difficult for him to return to the role of being a submissive student with the powerful teacher who has all the knowledge. Teaching methods that utilize an adult's self-directedness are more powerful.

5. A group of children in the second grade have probably had very similar life experiences to that point. However, as those children graduate from high school, mature, get jobs, and perhaps begin raising children, their life experiences begin to have a wide variation. When education is combined with these experiences it can be very rich and meaningful.

6. External factors such as a job promotion or career change motivate adult students. However, they can be even more motivated by internal factors such as self-esteem or job satisfaction (Knowles, Holton, & Swanson, 1998, pp. 64–68; Hancock, 2003, p. 15).

From the work of Malcolm Knowles, Stephen Lieb has identified six characteristics of adult learners:

1. "Adults are autonomous and self-directed." For that reason, the person being precepted should be included in developing objectives and desired learning outcomes. He/she should also assume responsibility for developing or finding some of the educational materials and presenting them to the preceptor.

2. "Adults have accumulated a foundation of life experiences and knowledge," which may be from work experience, other classes, volunteer activities, and family life. The education provided in the preceptor experience should build on these previous experiences and knowledge.

3. "Adults are goal oriented." Developing objectives and learning outcomes helps adult learners work with a preceptor to gain the knowledge and skills desired.

4. "Adults are relevancy oriented." Objectives and learning outcomes need to be related to the type of work the apprentice will be doing in the future.

5. "Adults are practical." Although understanding theories is important for adult learners, explaining how these theories relate to objectives, learning outcomes, and ultimately to the knowledge and skills the apprentice needs, is equally important.

6. Adults are not any different from other learners in that "they need to be shown respect." The preceptor needs to acknowledge the classroom and life experiences apprentices bring with them (Lieb, 1991).

TRANSFORMATIONAL LEARNING: CREATING MEANING FROM EXPERIENCE

For the development of guidelines for preceptors, the research on transformational learning adds to and complements the work by Knowles, providing direction in the creation of the learning experience. Baumgartner (2001) explains transformational learning in this way: "Knowledge is not 'out there' to be discovered but is created from interpretations and reinterpretations in light of new experiences" (p. 16). Transformational learning comes about when people create meaning from the experiences they have. It involves transforming or changing their perspective, habits, or way of thinking about something, leading to a modification in their frames of reference. By critically thinking about the assumptions they hold about something, talking with others who may have different ideas or beliefs, taking some action on their new insight, and finally evaluating the results, individuals change their frames of reference (Mezirow & Associates, 2000).

The steps used in the transformational learning process are to

1. help learners become aware of their own underlying assumptions
2. offer alternative theories and new assumptions
3. facilitate discourse either one-on-one or in a group setting
4. provide opportunities for critical reflection
5. move to further discourse (optional)
6. move to further critical reflection (optional)
7. have students express their new understanding through their new frame of reference (Hancock, 2003).

The points listed above are not necessarily sequential. For example, some discourse may actually occur first as the preceptor helps people discover assumptions they have. Some of the above points may also be repeated frequently during the process.

Teaching learners to become aware of their assumptions is probably the most difficult step to accomplish. The preceptor and apprentice may want to return to this point many times.

To facilitate discourse (the third point), it is necessary to establish a good professional relationship and a climate of trust. Without trust, it will be difficult to have a meaningful discussion about the assumptions a person holds and even more difficult to help with the transformation process.

There are many ways to develop trust between the preceptor and apprentice. Some are as simple as listening to the person, showing them through feedback that you understood what they were saying and then remembering their ideas so they can be incorporated at other times during the learning experience. It is also important to avoid blaming, ridiculing, or making broad generalizations. When a group is very diverse, cultural differences makes it difficult to tell jokes so that no one is offended. Of course, personal information must always be kept confidential. Finally, it is important to show respect for the students as adults because this respect develops into mutual trust. Showing respect includes consideration in developing assignments and then giving careful explanations of the assignments so that they do not appear to be busy work. The effort spent developing students' trust is important for a good educational experience.

GUIDELINES

From this brief overview of the work of these two researchers it is possible to develop some helpful guidelines for achieving a successful experience for the apprentice.

Guideline 1

The preceptor selected must be well prepared in the substantive content area and understand the characteristics of adult learners.

Based on the tenets of transformational learning, the role of the preceptor is to help the apprentice gain additional knowledge and skills in his/her area of expertise. If the preceptor is selected by a third party, that person needs a clear understanding of the abilities of both the preceptor and the apprentice to obtain a good fit between the two people. If the apprentice selects his/her own preceptor, he/she needs to understand the qualifications of the potential preceptors in order to achieve the educational experience desired.

Guideline 2

The preceptor and the apprentice must work together to develop the objectives and learning outcomes for the experience (Wlodkowski, 2001a).

There are four important components in this guideline.

1. Transformational learning concepts stress the importance of the preceptor's understanding the assumptions the apprentice brings to the experience. These assumptions provide the base on which the preceptor builds the learning experience. Usually a conversation based on a few questions such as "What do you hope to gain from this experience?" or "What are your major concerns?" will provide basic information. Another strategy is to modify a standard needs assessment test to fit the particular situation. No method will identify all of an apprentice's assumptions. As preceptors and apprentices work together and as a climate of trust and collegiality develops, the preceptor will find that the apprentice has other assumptions the preceptor may want to incorporate into the experience.

2. Knowles's work underscores the importance of the preceptor's understanding the goals the apprentice hopes to achieve from the experience so that, as much as possible, these goals can be incorporated into the experience. It is very easy to choose lofty goals with unrealistic expectations and so the preceptor will need to work with the apprentice so the apprentice understands how much can realistically be learned in one experience.

3. Objectives and desired learning outcomes must be clear and easily understood. Again, based on Knowles's work and the characteristics described by Lieb, the apprentice should understand how this experience will build on previous learning. Adult learners tend to be self-directed and can independently move ahead with the learning by reading professional journals, searching the Internet for related information, and so on (Wlodkowski, 2001a, 2001b).

4. Transformational learning can be enhanced when goals are stated as problem-solving goals. Wlodkowski explains that, "In working on a problem-solving goal, learners formulate or are given a problem to solve. Although the goal is clear (solve the problem) the learning is not definite or known beforehand" (Wlodkowski, 2001c, p. 158).

5. Finally, it is important for both the preceptor and the apprentice to have a mutual understanding about what will constitute a successful experience (Wlodkowski, 2001a).

Guideline 3

The learning environment is respectful to both the preceptor and the apprentice (Wlodkowski, 2001).

There are things the preceptor can do to establish a positive and respectful learning environment.

1. In most workplaces there are rules of conduct that professionals are expected to follow. If the apprentice is not or has not been employed in the same location as the preceptor these rules should be reviewed.

2. Transformational learning emphasizes dialogue and discussion. When the apprentice and the preceptor are from different cultures or backgrounds or have different first languages, it is important to acknowledge that words may have different meanings and that biases learned early in life need to be set aside.

In these circumstances preceptors may find it difficult to develop a good discussion or dialogue. One solution is to use a variation of Socratic questioning, not only to solve problems but also to better understand problems and the context in which they occur. This method involves identifying the instructional objective to be addressed and then planning a sequence of questions that will help the apprentice understand the concept. When this method is used, the preceptor should not be the only one asking the questions. The apprentice should also be encouraged to do so. Asking the apprentice to explain his/her understanding of the discussion helps ensure that there are no misunderstandings. Finally, summarizing the discussion is also beneficial (Hancock, 2003).

Guideline 4

Learning should move along a continuum from preceptor directed to apprentice directed (Hancock, 2003).

Immediately after objectives and learning outcomes are established, the preceptor should take the lead in directing learning activities. As the apprentice progresses through the preceptorship and see that his/her goals are being met by the learning experiences, the preceptor should encourage him/her to take more responsibility for his/her learning. This can be as simple as finding additional resources or as complex as developing a project related to the apprentices' area of interest.

Guideline 5

Learning should progress from beginning concepts to advanced ones (Hancock, 2003).

Organizing the learning experiences from simple to complex is also called assisted learning or scaffolding. This method involves "giving clues, information, prompts, reminders, and encouragement at the appropriate time and in the appropriate amount and then gradually allowing the [apprentice] to do more and more independently (Wlodkowski, 2001a). "Adults . . . appreciate the support assisted learning offers because it tends to be concrete, immediate and tailored to their . . . needs" (Wlodkowski, 2001a). Wlodkowski suggests several ways this can be done.

1. *Modeling* involves the preceptor demonstrating how to do something. The apprentice then performs the task under the supervision of the preceptor.

2. *Thinking out loud* is another method in which the preceptor states each step of the process needed to accomplish an activity.

3. *Anticipating difficulties* involves a discussion between the preceptor and the apprentice about where problems might occur and how they could be resolved.

4. The preceptor may also provide *prompts and/or cues* to help the apprentice remember the different steps required.

5. The *level of difficulty* of the activity can be *regulated* with easier tasks at the beginning and harder ones added as the apprentice gains proficiency.

6. *Reciprocal teaching* involves the apprentice teaching the preceptor a concept. This strategy works very well after the preceptor and apprentice have established a comfortable working rela-

tionship. Teaching someone else is an excellent way to reinforce a skill or concept.

7. Finally, *checklists* are helpful when there are many steps to remember (Wlodkowski, 2001a).

Guideline 6

Feedback is constructive and effective.

Prompt, constructive feedback is one of the most powerful tools a preceptor has to help the apprentice have a positive learning experience and outcome. Apprentices can "evaluate their progress . . . maintain their efforts toward realistic goals, self-assess, correct their errors efficiently, self-adjust and receive encouragement from instructors and others" (Wlodkowski, 2001b, p. 192). Some of the characteristics of effective feedback include:

1. *Providing sufficient information* to apprentices so that they understand the changes or modifications needed.

2. *Helping apprentices understand* how close they are to reaching the standard, objective, or goal, or how much more they need to do. For example, if giving professional presentations is a goal, the apprentice could be rated or scored on each of the attributes of an effective presentation.

3. *Being specific and constructive.* General suggestions do not help apprentices achieve their goals, but specific ones do. Preceptors should consider themselves successful if at the end of the educational experience apprentices can accurately assess their performance and adjust it according to the goal(s) they want to achieve.

4. *Providing timely feedback.* There may be situations when a delay in providing feedback is beneficial. For example, if the apprentice is very anxious or upset by the event, a delay will allow him/her time to calm down. The apprentice may better understand the feedback in a calmer state.

5. *Giving frequent feedback.* It is easier to correct a problem before a habit is firmly established or the situation is out of hand.

6. *Emphasizing good performances* and things done well rather than always focusing on problems.

7. Finally, *differential feedback*, which measures the difference between the prior feedback and the present, helps apprentices recognize how much they have improved in a specific skill. When trying to master difficult skills or concepts it is easy to be discouraged. Helping apprentices understand how much of a concept or skill they have mastered can provide the necessary encouragement to continue moving forward (Wlodkowski, 2001b).

The amount of feedback to provide is always a matter of judgment on the part of the preceptor. Too much feedback may cause apprentices to think they are incapable of any accomplishment, and too little feedback can lead them to think the preceptor is not interested. The middle ground will vary from apprentice to apprentice and may be difficult to find.

Guideline 7

The learning activities are relevant (Wlodkowski, 2001a).

Adult learners are busy people with multiple responsibilities. Activities included in this experience must be related to objectives and learning outcomes and apprentices need to understand how these activities relate to goals. Although there are many ways to ensure that this happens, there are two that are easy to use and that have stood the test of time. The first method uses the following five steps to create an interesting learning experience:

1. The activity is safe, so the apprentice will not feel embarrassed or humiliated if his/her performance is less than perfect.
2. The apprentice can be successful in some way with the activity.
3. The activity is interesting and not just "busy work." Adult learners with hectic lives are interested in projects or activities that hold their attention and relate to their learning objectives and outcomes; they are not motivated by projects that do not interest them.
4. There is some element of self-determination in the activity such as participation in a discussion or finding a journal article or Internet resource.
5. The activity is relevant for the apprentice. The preceptor may have selected the activity because of the apprentice's concerns, interests, or prior learning experiences (Wlodkowski, 2001).

The second method is called the K-W-L strategy and is composed of the following three phases:

Phase 1:   Learners identify what they think they **K**now about a specific topic (Wlodkowski, 2001b). Received by the preceptor in an accepting manner, this is a helpful way to uncover misconceptions and erroneous information about a specific topic.

Phase 2:   Learners find out what they **W**ould like to know about the topic. Questions and discussions during this phase provide opportunities for learning based upon apprentices' previous knowledge.

Phase 3:   What has been **L**earned is reviewed. This permits both the preceptor and the apprentice to evaluate the results of a particular activity (Wlodkowski, 2001).

Guideline 8

The assessments are fair, valid, and clear (Wlodkowski, 2001).

Assessment of activities, projects, and work of the apprentice by the preceptor is an important part of the learning experience. This assessment involves the evaluation of accomplishments. The criteria and methods by which the apprentice will be evaluated must be explained before the apprentice begins this learning experience. Assessment should be impartial and as free from cultural bias as possible. Exams and papers are only one way to evaluate the apprentice's performance. Demonstrations, the development of applications that can be used in future employment, and projects requiring the integrating of major concepts from different fields all provide meaningful assessments of learning that occurred during the preceptorship. If apprentices understand how they are to be evaluated they will be motivated to take more responsibility for their learning experience.

SUMMARY

Research and writing about adult learners is a good source of information for helping a person working as a preceptor develop an effective educational experience for an apprentice. From the research in the field of adult learning today, the work of two researchers, Malcolm Knowles, who focused on Andragogy, and Jack Mezirow, who studied Transformational Learning, were selected. These researchers provide a strong base for the eight guidelines that were discussed and that can be used in creating effective educational experiences for apprentices. The guidelines include: selecting preceptors well prepared in the substantive content area, the joint development of objectives and learning outcomes, a respectful learning environment, working toward an apprentice-centered environment, planning the educational experience so it moves from the simple to the complex, offering constructive feedback, using relevant learning activities, and having fair, valid, and clear assessments. Although other helpful guidelines could be used, the ones suggested here can help a preceptor create a valuable learning experience for an apprentice.

REFERENCES

Baumgartner, L. M. (2001). An update on transformational learning. In S. B. Merriam (Ed.), *The new update on adult learning theory* (pp. 15–24). San Francisco: Jossey-Bass.

Brookfield, S. D. (1986). *Understanding and facilitating adult learning*. San Francisco: Jossey-Bass.

Hancock, T. M. (2003). *ED 540: Adult education and self-directed learning, study guide*. Standish, ME: Saint Joseph's College.

Knowles, M. S., Holton, E. F., III, & Swanson, R. A. (1998). *The adult learner*. Woburn, MA: Butterworth-Heinemann.

Lieb, S. (1991, Fall). *Principles of adult learning VISION*. Retrieved March 2, 1998, from http://www.hcc.hawaii.edu/intranet/committees/FacDevCom/guidebk/teachtip/adults-2.htm

Merriam, S. B. (2001). Andragogy and self-directed learning: Pillars of adult learning theory. In S. B. Merriam (Ed.), *The new update on adult learning theory* (pp. 3–14). San Francisco: Jossey-Bass.

Merriam, S. B., & Brockett, R. G. (1997). *The profession and practice of adult education*. San Francisco: Jossey-Bass.

Merriam, S. B., & Caffarella, R. S. (2001). Andragogy and other models of adult learning. In S. B. Merriam, R. S. Caffarella, & P. Cranton (Eds.), *Adult learning, theories, principles and applications* (pp. 86–95). San Francisco: Jossey-Bass.

Mezirow, J., & Associates. (2000). *Learning as transformation*. San Francisco: Jossey-Bass.

Wlodkowski, R. J. (2001a). Helping adults develop positive attitudes toward learning. In S. B. Merriam, R. S. Caffarella, & P. Cranton (Eds.), *Adult learning, theories, principles and applications* (pp. 167–189). San Francisco: Jossey-Bass.

Wlodkowski, R. J. (2001b). Engendering competence among adult learners. In S. B. Merriam, R. S. Caffarella, & P. Cranton (Eds.), *Adult learning, theories, principles and applications* (pp. 190–214). San Francisco: Jossey-Bass.

Wlodkowski, R. J. (2001c). Establish inclusion among adult learners. In S. B. Merriam, R. S. Caffarella, & P. Cranton (Eds.), *Adult learning, theories, principles and applications* (pp. 145–164). San Francisco: Jossey-Bass.

SUGGESTED READING

Wilson, A. L., & Hayes, E. R. (Eds.). (2000). *The handbook of adult and continuing education*. San Francisco: Jossey-Bass.

CHAPTER 3

A Model Preceptor Program for Student Nurses

Deborah Wright Shpritz and Ann M. O'Mara

Nursing schools across the country are implementing inno-vative clinical courses and teaching strategies in response to changes in health care and nursing education. Despite increasing numbers of students applying to nursing schools, many schools cannot offer admission to all qualified students due to the decreasing numbers of clinical faculty and the decreasing availabil-ity of adequate clinical sites (American Association of Colleges of Nursing, 2004). This dilemma challenges faculty to find new approaches to clinical instruction. Until recently, the traditional approach to clinical teaching was one instructor supervising a group of 8–10 students. This approach creates a number of problems, including inadequate preparation of the student for the real world of nursing, insufficient time to practice complex technologies, and a superficial and unrealistic exposure to the complexities of the particular unit/facility. A number of nursing schools have discov-ered that this artificial reality ignores the immense contributions that experienced staff nurses can make to the student's full realiza-tion of nursing practice. Consequently, several nursing programs are using staff nurses as preceptors to help mitigate the reality shock often felt by the new graduate.

PURPOSE

The purpose of this chapter is to

1. describe preceptorships and the advantages and disadvantages of precepting undergraduate nursing students,
2. describe the roles and responsibilities of the involved individuals,
3. identify important factors in the selection process of faculty and preceptors,
4. describe the process of developing and implementing a preceptor course with reference to a model program, and
5. describe the process for designing and implementing a precepted course with reference to a model program.

PRECEPTOR PROGRAMS IN UNDERGRADUATE TEACHING

A preceptorship is a one-to-one contractual relationship between student and preceptor with a set time limit delineated at the beginning of the educational experience. The student works with the preceptor to achieve clearly defined professional, experiential objectives.

Often preceptorships are confused with apprenticeships, conjuring up the old diploma programs of the 20th century. Imbedded in the old concept of apprenticeship was the notion of contributing to the work environment with learning as a secondary outcome. With preceptorships, learning is and must be maintained as the primary goal. Accomplishing this goal involves a minimum of three individuals—the faculty member, the student, and the preceptor. The remainder of this chapter will use this simple triad as the exemplar for discussing all aspects of the preceptorship.

Whereas apprenticeships have a long and troubled history in nursing education, preceptorships are receiving positive evaluations in the contemporary world of nursing education. As early as 1981, Chickerella and Lutz maintained that the advantage of preceptorships outweighed the disadvantages. Just what are these advantages and disadvantages?

Advantages of Preceptor Programs to the Faculty

Serving as faculty for a precepted course does not abdicate the faculty's responsibility for educating and evaluating students. The advantages for faculty include flexibility, increased collegiality with other faculty and staff nurses in the clinical facility, and individualized time with students. Collaboration in research or continuing staff education is not only an advantage to the faculty, but may also serve as a reward to preceptors. With the continued emphasis on scholarly productivity in academic settings, access to patient populations for research is both important and problematic, especially in light of the HIPPA regulations. However, this access problem may be mitigated by the close working relationship that develops between faculty and preceptors. One outcome of this relationship can be the encouragement of staff by faculty to identify researchable clinical problems and ultimately to engage in collaborative research or other projects.

Unfortunately, the reality of staffing in most health care settings is often such that attending continuing education programs outside one's own facility is severely limited. Declining resources have also resulted in reduced professional development staff formerly available to provide individualized continuing education programs to clinical staff. Faculty members are well prepared to assist in the preparation and presentation of relevant clinical topics either in a lecture in-service format, journal club, or by conducting nursing grand rounds. Faculty can also serve as a resource for preceptors, the clinical unit, and the education department.

Advantages of Preceptor Programs to the Preceptor

A number of advantages and sources of satisfaction have been identified in the literature. In fact, these sources of satisfaction have often been the impetus for clinical agencies to seek collaborative relationships, in the form of preceptorships, with schools of nursing. The most notable advantage is increased job satisfaction. Related to this general feeling of satisfaction is the fact that preceptors find that teaching students

1. adds a new dimension to their work worlds, keeping them challenged and stimulated and increasing their level of professionalism;

2. affords different kinds of teaching opportunities that can influence nursing practice;
3. motivates them to maintain and upgrade clinical skills and knowledge;
4. affords opportunities to learn from students; and
5. contributes to professional growth and development and promotion.

In addition to the advantages for the preceptor, there are advantages for nursing service/education. As students' performance can be closely scrutinized, recruiting new graduates takes on a different dimension. Nurse managers recognize that orientation of new graduates who have precepted on their assigned unit is accomplished more efficiently and effectively. This process enhances new employees' transition to their role as nurses.

Advantages of Preceptor Programs to the Student

In general, nursing educators agree that using preceptorships in nursing education, particularly in the students' final semester, can build students' confidence and self-esteem, increase the level of independent functioning, provide opportunities for role socialization and for acquisition of competence and confidence in performing clinical and problem-solving skills, critical thinking, and the application of theory to practice (DeYoung, 2003; Gaberson & Oermann, 1999; Oermann, 1996).

On a more practical level, students find their learning needs are more easily met and their anxieties reduced. They have learned how to demonstrate their skills and knowledge to potential employers. Having their eyes opened to the reality of professional nursing practice is a maturing experience for most students; they get to experience the typical day of a nurse. Students learn better time management and organizational skills, as well as the importance of flexibility. Such comments as, "I had no idea nursing was so multifaceted," "Nursing is more teamwork than I thought," and "What I was taught in class really is relevant!" demonstrate the tremendous growth nursing students experience when precepted. Students also show increased responsibility for their own learning, setting the stage for lifelong learning.

Haas, Deardorff, Klotz, and colleagues (2002) identified unanticipated benefits for students in a precepted experience. Percepted students were found to be able to assume more responsibility, prioritize more acutely ill patients, and perform a greater number of skills than students in a nonprecepted course. Camaraderie developed between the student and preceptor. Students felt a sense of inclusion on the unit and became more actively involved in seeking information from a variety of sources (e.g., preceptor, physician, literature) and sharing it with faculty.

Disadvantages of Preceptor Programs to the Faculty

Whereas many may think being the faculty in a precepted course is easy and not as labor intensive as teaching in a regular classroom or being an on-site clinical instructor, a precepted course does have its disadvantages. The evaluation process can produce a number of anxieties for faculty. If the preceptor's information on student behaviors is incomplete or vague, an adversarial relationship can arise between preceptor and student.

Instead of the usual one-to-nine student ratio, faculty now deal with a preceptor for every student. Student numbers may approach 20 in a course. That means the faculty must interact with 40 people, not including the nurse managers who are often the starting point of the preceptorship process. Site visits and follow-up phone calls to preceptors and students are extremely time consuming. Because most preceptors prefer not to be called at home, contacting them during work hours can be difficult, as preceptors often change shifts.

Faculty must be reachable when students are on the clinical units. This on-call status can be stressful and demanding. Making site visits to different clinical facilities can also be demanding and time consuming, especially if facilities are not in close proximity to one another. Additionally, it is sometimes difficult to find time to talk with students during site visits to the unit due to unit activities, the patient's condition, or the student's increased involvement in unit activities.

In general, the academic semester defines the beginning and the ending to courses. Unfortunately, this may not be the case with precepted courses. Faculty spend more time organizing and preparing for a precepted course. Several weeks to a month prior to the start of the course, faculty must spend a considerable amount of time negotiating student placements and orienting preceptors. Even after a relationship is established with a clinical facility or unit, it is not safe to assume that the same unit and preceptor will be available for each subsequent semester. Thus, the negotiating process is ongoing.

Despite the identified disadvantages to all members of the relationship, preceptorships in undergraduate nursing programs are flourishing (Bain, 1996; Haas et al., 2002; Lengacher & Tittle, 2000; McCarty & Higgins, 2003; Trevitt, Grealish, & Reaby, 2001). Although most programs are using preceptors to bridge the ideal of the educational environment with the reality of the workplace, the literature identifies use of the preceptorship model at different places in the curriculum (Beeman, 2001; Nordgren, Richardson, & Laurella, 1998) and in a variety of settings (Lengacher & Tittle). In this chapter, the focus will be on preceptorships used in the students' final semester.

Disadvantages to the Preceptor

Release time from usual patient assignments for preceptoring is seldom an option, and preceptors must determine how they will blend patient care with student teaching. For some, this is a challenging and satisfying art but for others, it is a source of frustration and stress. Inadequate preparation and inexperienced staff (less than 1 year) are additional difficulties. Without rewards and/or support, preceptor burnout can occur. This is especially the case if the same preceptor is continually used semester after semester. Balancing the complex needs of patients with the learning needs of students is the major challenge for the preceptor. The increasing complexity of patient care and decreased length of stay of many patients can also be seen as a drawback. This balancing act usually translates into extra time spent and increased responsibility at work.

Disadvantages of Preceptor Programs to the Student

Usually the advantages of the precepted experience outweigh the disadvantages. However, it is important that students be aware of the potential disadvantages. Prior student experience in the clinical setting has usually been limited in terms of daily clinical hours.

Teaming with preceptors requires students to work the same shift, which can be 12 hours long. Often students are not prepared for these long days. Students with this difficulty are advised to gradually increase their workdays from 8 hours to 10 hours to 12 hours to ease the transition.

Students must also balance course schedules with preceptors' work schedules. Factoring in family time and time to complete course assignments and scheduling the required number of hours can sometimes be difficult. Additionally, clinical time can potentially be canceled if the preceptor is ill or if his/her schedule is changed unexpectedly.

Working on a specific unit for the precepted course confines students' experience to one patient population. Students' opportunity to practice skills is limited to those associated with the unit, which can be limiting when applying for a job following graduation.

Evaluation Process

Students may find the evaluation process more difficult than the usual clinical grading process, particularly those who are in danger of failing. Instead of the usual faculty–student relationship governing the evaluation process, now there is a third person (the preceptor) involved in the relationship. Faculty seldom directly observe student behaviors; rather they rely on the preceptors' observations and, based on these observations, judge the students' ability or inability to accomplish clinical objectives.

Preceptee–Preceptor Relationship

Work expectations and communication styles may be a source of friction in the preceptee–preceptor relationship. What preceptors expect students to accomplish and learn may not be congruent with students' expectations or may even be beyond their capabilities.

Preceptor Absences

There are times, due to illness or other commitments, when the preceptor will be absent and another staff member must fill in as the student's preceptor. Just as students find it hard to rotate from one clinical site to another, similar anxieties and uncertainties arise when the preceptor is absent. This is particularly true when the preceptee–preceptor relationship is a strong, mutually rewarding one. However, some students have viewed this occurrence as an opportunity to see alternative problem-solving and communication styles and different methods of organizing the workday.

ROLES AND RESPONSIBILITIES: FACULTY, PRECEPTORS, STUDENTS

The potential success of any precepted relationship relies on a clear understanding of the roles and responsibilities of all involved individuals. The following discussion highlights the major responsibilities of each member.

Faculty Role

Lambert and Lambert (2001) identify faculty roles as those of consultant and coevaluator. Faculty in a precepted experience must facilitate relationships between preceptors and students, monitor student learning experiences, and evaluate student performance. Facilitating the experience is the most critical as it requires faculty to be clear and open communicators. Validation, rephrasing, and summarizing conversations with preceptors should be done frequently. When discussing the clinically weak student with the preceptor, faculty may need to follow up and write formal summaries. Successful facilitation of the relationship will aid in faculty monitoring and evaluating students' progress.

The work of Hseih and Knowles (1990) summarizes the relevant issues related to the faculty role in facilitating the preceptorship relationship and ultimately monitoring and evaluating students. Hseih and Knowles identify seven themes as important to the preceptorship relationship:

1. Faculty are the catalysts for building and maintaining *trust* with preceptors and students, as well as between students and preceptors.
2. By clearly defining expectations of all participants faculty can greatly reduce confusion among participants. Handouts, a course description, and a preceptor manual are helpful in reinforcing expectations.

3. The usual set of *support systems* is no longer in place for either the preceptor (coworkers are not often preceptors) or the student (peers who may not be on the same unit). The faculty's role is to encourage preceptors and students to verbalize concerns, problems, and the changed roles associated with preceptorships.

4. Just as all students do not come with prerequisite skills and knowledge, not all preceptors possess requisite teaching and communication skills. *Honestly communicating* the potential for less than perfect performance to both the preceptor and student sets the stage for a positive experience. By implementing this approach early in the relationship, faculty can avoid the pitfalls inherent in 3-person interactions.

5. The manner in which one learns must be *respected and accepted*. The classic counterexample of this is the strict and regimented training of earlier schools of nursing in comparison to the present approach using adult learning principles. Faculty must take the lead in helping students understand preceptors' teaching methods, and, conversely, helping preceptors understand students' approach to learning. The goal is to reach consensus and not threaten anyone's basic personality.

6. Acknowledging feelings of uncertainty and anxiety on the part of both the preceptor and student will go a long way in maintaining everyone's sense of self-worth. Such techniques as self-disclosure, positive feedback, and an attitude of confidence will facilitate an environment of *encouragement*.

7. Faculty successful in implementing the above aspects of a preceptor program will require a considerable amount of *mutual sharing of self and experience* between preceptor and student. Closely related to this is the sense of trust that faculty must convey to the preceptor and the student.

Evaluation of Students

In the grading of clinical performance, Pass/Fail grades facilitate identifying student behaviors and evaluating student performance. Only faculty have the requisite skills and knowledge of the evaluation process for deciding student achievement of course objectives. Emphasizing that this responsibility remains with faculty can considerably reduce a preceptor's anxiety. On more than one occasion a preceptor has said, "I don't want the responsibility of deciding this student's fate." Although the preceptor plays a large role in the decision-making process, the final decision and its communication to the student rests with faculty. Two issues regarding evaluating students include explaining to the preceptor that it actually is the faculty who determines the student's grade and handling those students who are unsafe, lack adequate knowledge, or act unprofessionally.

From initial meetings with preceptors, faculty must continually emphasize the preceptor's role in describing student behaviors. The next step involves giving faculty interpretation of student behavior feedback to the preceptor. For example, when a preceptor is unsure as to the safety of a student's actions (e.g., using correct techniques, stating accurate rationale), faculty must obtain specific clinical examples, including a time frame, and explain to the preceptor how these actions are (or are not) meeting clinical objectives.

It goes without saying that some students will not be successful, be it in a traditional or a precepted clinical experience. When such situations arise, before concluding that the student is not successfully meeting objectives, faculty must closely scrutinize the setting, including the preceptor. The following situation illustrates this point.

"I Had No Idea I Was Anxious."

Laura's first choice for her precepted experience was the ICU. In addition to being experienced, her preceptor was a warm, nurturing individual who did everything in her power to help students be successful. She recognized the complexities of the ICU and was able to provide rich learning experiences. On the faculty's first visit to the unit, nonverbal behaviors of frustration with Laura on the part of the preceptor were observed; however, the level of acuity in the unit precluded any in-depth discussion with the preceptor. Laura, on the other hand, appeared calm as she followed the preceptor everywhere.

The faculty's follow-up conversation revealed a disturbing situation. Although Laura's nonverbal behavior indicated calmness, her conversations with the preceptor and other staff members suggested otherwise. For example, on a particularly busy day when one staff member had called in sick, Laura insisted on going to lunch and belittled the staff for not doing the same. When the preceptor reminded Laura of how busy the unit was and how potentially unsafe it could be, Laura responded that she had not thought of it in that way. On several occasions, Laura was late arriving, or asked to go home early. Despite the preceptor's and the faculty's spelling out for Laura the inappropriateness of her behavior, it continued.

At the conclusion of the fifth clinical day, with eight more remaining, the preceptor could see no significant improvement in Laura's professional demeanor and believed she could no longer be an effective preceptor to this student. Given that Laura had no previous record of such behavior, the faculty considered other factors, especially the chaotic nature of the ICU. The faculty member called Laura into her office, reviewed the sequence of events, and told her she was removing her from this clinical setting. When the faculty member explored the environment and Laura's desire to be placed in the ICU, two issues emerged. The motivation to work in the ICU was not entirely Laura's, as she felt compelled to follow the trend of her peers. Many of her friends praised the ICU because "there is much more there to learn." In the final analysis, Laura really thought that there was an equal amount to be gained by working on a general medical-surgical unit.

The second issue was that the ICU setting posed unforeseen problems for Laura. This particular ICU was located in the cancer center of the medical facility. Less than a year prior to the experience, Laura's father had died of acute leukemia. She had watched him succumb to the complications of sepsis and respiratory failure. During her 5 days in the ICU, the majority of patients were being treated for one or both of these medical problems. In exploring these aspects, the faculty posed the idea that perhaps Laura had considerable anxiety. At first Laura denied her feelings, but later recognized that her insomnia and loss of appetite might also be related.

Laura was placed on a step-down coronary care unit with the understanding that without significant improvement in her professional behavior she would fail the course. By the third clinical day in the new environment, Laura was proving to be a mature, highly self-directed student. She successfully met the course objectives and the second preceptor did not observe any unprofessional behaviors.

Although many aspects of this scenario are positive, faculty regretted the fact that the first preceptor did not want to have anything to do with Laura after her removal from the ICU. In the faculty's conference with Laura, the student posed the question of going to the preceptor and apologizing for her behavior. Instead she was advised to write a letter to the preceptor, outlining what had occurred. Under a different set of circumstances, the faculty believes the preceptor would have seen a very different student.

In situations where a student is clearly unsafe, the implementation of school policies and procedures related to unsafe performance should be followed. Due process is essential, with all evaluative statements emanating from the faculty, not the preceptor.

Preceptor Role

Broadly speaking, the role of the preceptor is to bridge the gap between the idealism of the academic environment and the reality of the workplace. The preceptor role is one of the most effective in bridging this gap. Lambert and Lambert (2001) see the roles of the preceptor as teacher/role model, workplace socializer, and coevaluator. Through role modeling, coaching, demonstration, and dialogue, the preceptor helps the student ease the transition to the "real" world of nursing (Rittman & Osburn, 1995). Preceptors can help guide students through problem solving and the critical thinking process by thinking out loud when they make decisions regarding patient care. Preceptors often say they feel uncomfortable and silly doing this as they just do it automatically. After providing an explanation to the preceptor as to the value of this exercise, most are willing to try it. Anecdotal student feedback indicates that it is most helpful.

Above all else, honest and open communication will establish a positive learning environment. The following responsibilities are germane to the preceptor role. The preceptor should

1. contract with the student for a specific period of time for the clinical experiences during the semester and provide an orientation to the clinical unit,
2. collaborate with the student to develop learning experiences congruent with the student's goals and objectives,

3. provide specific and effective ongoing feedback to the student through verbal and written communication,
4. communicate with faculty as to the student's progress and the nature of his or her overall learning experience,
5. be open to the need to change and grow, and
6. never abandon the student.

Unfortunately, many of these responsibilities are added to the numerous patient and unit responsibilities of the preceptor. Adequate preparation is an effective means for helping preceptors identify strategies for balancing these multiple demands.

Student Role

The student's role in a precepted course is that of learner and collaborator (Lambert & Lambert, 2001). With a full understanding of the course and clinical objectives, students will be formulating individualized learning objectives. Unlike the traditional clinical course, the student will be sharing these objectives with an additional individual, the preceptor. Individualized attention from the preceptor and faculty can help students formulate and revise learning objectives. Who has more knowledge of the rich learning opportunities available on the unit than the preceptor? For students who have some difficulty identifying individual objectives, working a couple of shifts on the unit with the preceptor can give them a more concrete idea of the patient population and the learning opportunities available to them. The student's role is to tap into this wealth of information. The following situation describes these advantages.

Learning Opportunities

For many years, faculty have supervised students in the traditional manner of bringing a group of 8–10 students onto a general medical-surgical unit and providing as many learning experiences as possible. Although faculty required each student to write individualized goals, the accomplishment of these goals was constrained by time (i.e., presence on the unit restricted to Thursdays and Fridays), patient availability (i.e., unit capacity of 24 beds), and staffing patterns. Observing a cardiac catheterization was not an option because it was only done on Mondays and Wednesdays. Most, if not all, students wrote psychomotor learning goals related to parenteral medications or sterile procedures. At the conclusion of the semester, it was not unusual for some students to have missed the opportunity for one or more of these experiences. A course using preceptors changes all of that.

In the process of creating and piloting a required precepted course, faculty have no idea of the extent of learning opportunities that will become available to students. The logistics of the course require the student to spend 126 hours over 7 weeks with a preceptor in a selected area of interest. These 126 hours average approximately 18 hours per week; however, faculty caution students not to confine themselves in this manner. Rather, the objective is to show 126 hours of clinical time at the end of 7 weeks (some weeks may be 24 hours, other weeks 8 hours). Students are expected to negotiate with preceptors and fit the hours in around their other school class times. Consequently, students may spend an occasional weekend with the preceptor, and, often, students are never in the clinical area on the same 2 days in successive weeks.

Flexibility in scheduling, coupled with the lack of competition for learning activities on the unit (usually only one or two students are precepted on any one unit) opens a number of doors to the student. For example: a Cancer Center, consisting of two medical units, a surgical unit, an ICU, and an ambulatory clinic, was one of the first to become involved in the course and provided a wonderful example of that wealth of learning opportunities. When students were precepted on one of the oncology units, they were offered the following opportunities as part of their total clinical experience: observational days on the other units as well as in surgery, observing one of the ongoing support groups, and participation in any of the core oncology courses offered to the staff. Because there were only one or two students on the unit, the entire staff became vested in the students' learning, offering multiple opportunities to observe and practice complex procedures.

Once the door to learning had been opened, students, on the whole, became eager and creative in identifying other learning opportunities. For example, several students became involved in the data collection of a faculty member's ongoing study of coping in cancer patients.

Self-direction is a quality faculty look for and demand of all students; it is a must in a preceptorship. The advantage in a preceptorship is the support faculty can often gain from the preceptor in encouraging students to be self-directed. Often students are shocked when they find that they are expected to devise their own clinical schedules. For some this first assignment is problematic. Students have available to them information regarding the flexibility of their clinical days and are advised that they may be expected to work weekends and off shifts with their preceptors. When given this information early, students are usually able and willing to make the necessary changes in their lives and schedules.

Another aspect of self-direction is accountability. Prior to the precepted course students are held accountable by required preclinical preparation time, thereby giving them the time and opportunity to acquire the necessary knowledge and skills for safe practice. The precepted course usually is the first one for which students cannot prepare ahead of time. Last semester seniors need to be exposed to situations where they must effectively and efficiently obtain essential information for safe practice in the work setting. Preparation must be defined differently in a preceptorship. The knowledge the student brings is not as important as the student's accountability in finding the answers. From the start, faculty tell students that the statement, "I don't know" must be followed with "but I will look it up before (giving the medication, doing the procedure)." Consequently, most students bring a number of references to their clinical sites, either personal digital assistants (PDAs) such as a Palm or Handspring Visor containing relevant drug references, or drug calculation tools and calculators, general nursing resources, journal articles, and nursing texts.

Assertiveness is another facet of self-direction that faculty need to require and nurture in students. Often students are placed in somewhat passive roles in the traditional clinical setting. They are competing for limited learning opportunities and a certain amount of luck determines whether they will be selected for a particular one. Because this opportunity is greatly reduced in preceptorships, students must consistently articulate their learning needs to their preceptors. Experienced preceptors are often adept in helping students identify and accomplish selected learning goals. Students working with new preceptors may need some guidance to remind the preceptor what it is they want from the experience.

THE SELECTION PROCESS

A process of selecting individuals for a precepted course should be considered for all three members of the preceptorship relationship. The following discussion highlights some of the more important issues to consider.

Selecting the Faculty

Length of teaching experience and the ability to delegate student supervision are the two most important criteria in selecting faculty to teach a precepted course. Generally speaking, faculty lacking these attributes are not well suited to manage a precepted course. Faculty relinquish control of the clinical learning experience; direct supervision is delegated to the preceptor. Often, less experienced faculty have some difficulty with this lack of control. Related activities, such as asking students about their preparation, identifying appropriate patient assignments, and observing student–patient interactions, are not part of the faculty role in this model.

Selecting Preceptors

Considerable control can be exercised when selecting preceptors. Lambert and Lambert (2001) identify three groups of characteristics to be considered in deciding whether someone should be a preceptor: clinical nursing characteristics, professional characteristics, and personality characteristics.

Clinical nursing characteristics include at least 1 year of clinical experience, comprehensive knowledge, and interest in professional growth and mastery of clinical skills. When considering the nurse's *length of experience in a particular specialty*, explore where the experience has been. For example, a nurse with 5 years medical-surgical experience, but who is new (i.e., less than 1 year) to the field of neuroscience, may not be the best candidate for a neuroscience preceptorship.

Assess the nurse's work schedule to determine whether it will fit with the student's school schedule. Although a number of part-time staff display many attributes of a good preceptor, unless they work at least 30 hours each week, the student will have difficulty acquiring the necessary time to achieve course objectives. A variation on this is the weekend-alternative staff. Given the increasing diversity of students, the weekend-alternative clinical experience may be very appealing, for example, to students with small children.

Professional characteristics of a good preceptor include excellent leadership skills, outstanding communication skills, good decision-making skills, advocacy for the learner, and the ability to use resources effectively. A *recommendation from the preceptor's immediate supervisor* regarding these skills should be sought. Teaching experience is helpful but not always a realistic expectation.

When considering the potential preceptor's credentials, many state boards of nursing stipulate that preceptors must possess the minimum of a bachelor's degree in nursing in order to precept an undergraduate baccalaureate student. Oulette (1993) found that students who were precepted by baccalaureate-prepared nurses had greater professional socialization than those who were not. Additionally certification in one's subspecialty, such as oncology (i.e., Oncology Nursing Society), critical care (i.e., American Association for Critical Care Nurses Certification Corporation), or neurosciences (American Board of Neuroscience Nursing) indicates a commitment to professional development.

Desirable personality characteristics include patience and enthusiasm; a nonthreatening and nonjudgmental attitude toward others; a flexible, open-minded, trustworthy manner; a sense of humor; self-confidence; willingness to share knowledge and skills; and willingness to commit the time involved in being a preceptor. Of all these, the most important is the willingness and desire to be a preceptor, particularly in light of declining resources available for rewarding the role (Manager's Forum, 2001).

In the majority of cases, no monetary payment is made to the preceptor for assuming the role; recognition is the reward. The incentive to be a preceptor may be the opportunity to work one-on-one with a student to influence his/her nursing practice. Some schools offer other small tokens as rewards to preceptors including library privileges, tuition waivers, recognition luncheons or dinners, attendance at continuing education conferences, or special title designations. Agencies may reward preceptors by providing special meals, supplying money to attend conferences, or integrating the role into a clinical ladder for promotional purposes (Manager's Forum, 2001). It is up to the school of nursing and the agency to negotiate rewards or incentives for preceptors. For many, being valued is actually more important than monetary compensation.

Student Selection

Students cannot be selected for a precepted course based on credentials or other attributes, particularly if it is a required course. Rather than a selection process, students undergo an education or orientation process to the precepted course and the roles of the preceptor and preceptee. A preceptee will often be the only student on the unit, and finding immediate support from peers may not be easy. When there is considerable latitude in placement students' input may help alleviate the sense of isolation they often feel while on the unit.

DESIGNING AND IMPLEMENTING A PRECEPTED COURSE

With the full understanding of the roles and responsibilities of the faculty, student, and preceptor, faculty should find designing a precepted course similar to designing a traditional clinical course. In fact, any clinical course can use preceptors. Much depends on the role faculty wish the preceptors to play in the course. The course described here requires the student to synthesize previously learned material and to develop a personal philosophy of nursing. A preceptorship plays a critical role in helping the student meet these requirements.

Placement in the Curriculum

The course described here, the Senior Clinical Practicum, is the student's final clinical course before graduation, with all courses in the program being either pre- or corequisites to the practicum. The course is described in extremely broad terms, thus allowing student placements in a variety of settings. Students have been placed in such diverse settings as ambulatory clinics, school-based clinics, rehabilitation facilities, and long-term care facilities. Students are encouraged to identify their own placements preferences.

POLICIES AND PROCEDURES

Even the most self-directed, mature students need some structure. In designing the precepted course, having policies and procedures in place helps provide structure. Policies, procedures and guidelines should be congruent with those of the academic institution and the clinical agency. Tables 3.1 and 3.2 list some of the policies, procedures, and scheduling guidelines for a precepted course.

Grading Policies

Clinical objectives are usually Pass/Fail; all objectives are derived from earlier courses. Clinical objectives must be attainable in all settings and, therefore, are stated in very broad terms. The student is evaluated in the following areas: professional development, nurse–patient relationship, assimilation as a member of the health care team, and the nursing process: assessment, analysis, planning, implementation, and evaluation. Students must earn a "Pass" in the clinical component in order to receive a passing grade for the total course.

In addition to the clinical component, a weekly seminar provides the didactic component of the course and yields its overall letter grade. Students are graded on their seminar attendance and participation and completion of written assignments, including a case study presentation of a patient of their choosing whom they have cared for on the clinical unit. The weekly seminar is also a venue for discussing students' professional development and designing individual plans for directing their career in nursing. This includes graduate study, the value of professional organizations, résumé writing, and developing a study plan for passing NCLEX.

Clinical Sites

Prior to the semester in which the precepted course is to be offered, faculty begin the process of identifying potential clinical sites for students. This selection can be done through personal communications of faculty and the agency's education department or through letters sent to agencies that have a clinical affiliation with the school of nursing. Faculty have found that personal communication works best to ascertain if the agency is unable to participate because

TABLE 3.1   Clinical Policies and Procedures: Student Responsibilities

---

1. Students must participate in a unit orientation.
2. A clinical schedule must be submitted to the faculty with each new work schedule. Faculty must approve clinical schedules and all changes in clinical schedules. Hours not approved are subject to "make up" time. If the proposed work schedule must be changed, faculty must be notified prior to the schedule change.
3. All student assignments must be coassigned with the student's preceptor. As the preceptor is ultimately responsible for the care given to patients, regular assessment and follow-up of student's performance is expected.
4. Some facilities require that any student signature needs to be cosigned by the preceptor as part of the end-of-shift routine.
5. All incident reports involving the student or the student's patients need to be cosigned by the preceptor, and faculty must be notified.
6. Students must be supervised for **all medications** being given. Some agencies may limit the medications that students can give. Students must adhere to the agency policy as it relates to student administration of medications.
7. Students should be supervised for all invasive procedures (e.g., suctioning, catheterization, etc.) by the preceptor.
8. Primary care is to be provided only to the assigned patient(s). However, supervised observations of other patients on the unit can occur at the discretion of the preceptor.
9. Students who are reporting absent must call the unit, leave a message for the preceptor with the charge nurse, and notify the faculty member at least 1 hour prior to the clinical experience. Any clinical time missed must be made up under the supervision of the preceptor or an approved substitute.
10. **Illness or Injury:** Students should be referred to student health during daytime hours or to the emergency room when working evenings or nights. Faculty should be notified as soon as possible.
11. **When Preceptor is Ill:** Another preceptor may be assigned to work with the student so that the work schedule as originally designed by the student and the preceptor can be maintained. An alternative experience can also be arranged if possible (e.g., Operating Room or Cardiac Catheterization observation).
12. Students are expected to arrive at least 15 minutes before the start of the clinical shift.
13. Students scheduling night clinical work must verify **safe** transportation to and from the clinical agency.
14. All written assignments must be submitted to faculty on time. Faculty will grade assignments and return them to students during the next class meeting.
15. Students are **required** to attend all seminar sessions of the course as scheduled by faculty.
16. Midterm and final clinical evaluations will be conducted formally by faculty. Students are responsible for self-evaluation at this time.
17. If students are not prepared or need remediation, faculty will assist these students. Preceptors should notify faculty as soon as possible so that students can be removed from the clinical area and remediation can begin.

(continued)

TABLE 3.1 *(continued)*

18. Students who show deficiencies during the rotation must meet with the faculty member to outline areas for improvement and should meet each clinical day to review and document progress.
19. **Dress Code:** Students should wear the official school of nursing uniform unless an exception is authorized by faculty. School of nursing identification badges must be worn at all times. Some agencies may require an additional identification badge specific to their institution. Students must also adhere to the agency dress code involving hair, piercings, shoes, jewelry, and so forth.
20. Students need to take responsibility for learning and must seek guidance as appropriate.
21. **Safety and Honesty:** Students are to refer to the academic institution's student handbook regarding the policy on "Unsafe Clinical Performance of Nursing Students" and "Academic Dishonesty and Irregularity."

TABLE 3.2 Policies and Procedures for Student-Initiated Clinical Placements

1. Students may not be precepted by a family member or personal acquaintance.
2. In general, students may not be precepted on a unit where they are currently employed. In rare circumstances, with full cooperation and understanding from the nurse manager, a student may be precepted on the unit, but it must be on a shift that the student does not normally work.
3. To be a preceptor, a staff nurse must have a minimum of a baccalaureate degree in nursing and at least 1 year experience as a registered nurse.
4. If the student has a particular preceptor in mind, he or she is to forward to the course coordinator, in writing, at least 1 month prior to the first day of class, the following information:
   a. Name of preceptor, credentials, years of experience;
   b. Clinical facility, type of unit, unit phone number;
   c. Name and phone number of preceptor's first-line supervisor (usually this is the nurse manager); and
   d. Name and phone number of the director of staff development, or the equivalent person in charge of student placement in the particular unit.
5. If the student has a particular clinical facility in mind but not a preceptor, he or she is to forward to the course coordinator, in writing, at least 1 month prior to the first day of class, the following information:
   a. Name and phone number of the clinical facility; and
   b. Name and phone number of the director of staff development or the equivalent person in charge of student placements in the facility.

of internal policies (e.g., faculty must be on-site, no unlicensed precepted students) or staffing restrictions. Additionally, placement of students in acute care settings is often complicated by decreased length of stay for patients in acute care facilities, affecting occupancy rates and the nursing shortage. Identifying alternative clinical sites such as home health agencies, long-term care facilities, and community settings is also important. For some students, the large academic health center is overwhelming and unfriendly. Small, community-based, and rural hospitals can be ideal placements for these students.

Students are asked during preregistration to complete a "Clinical Preference Questionnaire" to help faculty make appropriate placements. Information includes the students preference for clinical specialties (e.g., adult, pediatrics, community health) and subspecialties (e.g., neuroscience, critical care, oncology), any transportation difficulties, geographical preferences, and employment information.

As faculty become more experienced with a precepted course, students can be given an increasing amount of freedom to find their own clinical placements. Table 3.2 describes the process for a student-initiated clinical placement. Some facilities, particularly those used by a number of different nursing programs, have requested only faculty contact for student placements. Smaller, less frequently used facilities have embraced the notion of working with students to find a suitable placement. By giving students this freedom there is less pressure on faculty to contact so many facilities. Faculty have also found that students who establish their own sites are more enthusiastic about the experience.

PRECEPTOR PREPARATION

Preparation of the preceptor for the role of clinical teacher is as important as preparing the student for the precepted experience. The method of preparation varies, depending on the school of nursing and the clinical agency. A preceptor workshop is preferable, where there can be face-to-face interaction of preceptors and faculty. The reality of today's health care environment is that the in-person attendance of a preceptor at a workshop is not always feasible. Some agencies offer a preceptor workshop twice yearly, inviting all nurses who are interested in becoming preceptors to attend (Meng & Conti, 1995). One-on-one orientation of the preceptor may also be required, especially at smaller agencies where only one or two students are placed. Regardless of which method of preparing the preceptor is used, the following topics should be included:

1. curriculum overview and course description;
2. roles of faculty, student, and preceptor;
3. adult learning principles;
4. teaching strategies;
5. legal ramifications of precepting an unlicensed student;
6. methods of describing student performance versus evaluating student performance; and,
7. chronology of student progression so that preceptors have an indication of where students should be at various points in the experience.

Curriculum Overview and Course Description

It is important that preceptors understand how the precepted course fits into the overall education of the student. Course description, objectives, requirements, evaluation of student performance, and policies and procedures are discussed.

Roles: Faculty, Student, Preceptor

Preceptors are given essentially the same information on roles that was presented earlier in this chapter. Preceptors usually have a number of questions related to role delineation. Most frequently asked questions relate to the use of faculty by the preceptor and under what circumstances the student is held (or not held) accountable.

Preceptors are told to call faculty when they believe it is essential to remove the student from the clinical unit for whatever reason, when they think that student behavior needs to be validated, and any time they feel they need to communicate with faculty. When in doubt or if preceptors *think* they should call the faculty for something, preceptors should call.

Teaching Strategies and the Adult Learner

Whereas all nurses are educated to and have assumed the role of teacher, the preceptors' perspective is often limited to patients. The goal of preceptor preparation is to broaden that perspective. This can be done by having guest speakers review case scenarios and by asking participants to reflect on their own educational experiences. Videotaping guest speakers can be valuable for future workshops or for those participants who cannot attend.

A discussion of the phenomena that can affect the teaching–learning environment is important. In addition to the obvious ones of patients' emotional responses, presence of other health care providers, and changes in patient status, preceptors also learn and are encouraged to include strategies such as role-playing and problem solving using case studies. Other important topics include conflict management, role modeling, and effective ways to motivate students.

Describing Student Performance versus Evaluating Student Performance

Although the roles of the preceptor and faculty are delineated, special consideration is given to a more thorough exploration of student evaluations. Preceptors often express confusion and anxiety with regard to this process. A number of clinical examples can be used to reinforce their role. Another concern of faculty are those preceptors who are unable to tell a student his/her weaknesses and yet express to the faculty serious reservations regarding the student's abilities for safe practice. Due process is an important theme during the presentation of this topic. The need to keep both student and faculty apprised of student performance is emphasized. The relationship between student performance and achieving clinical objectives is also emphasized.

Legal Ramifications to Precepting Unlicensed Students

The best speaker for this topic is a nurse educator who is also a lawyer. Using the state's Nurse Practice Act as the framework, the speaker presents a review of the concepts of negligence, malpractice, and legal accountability as they relate to the Nurse Practice Act and precepting. Several legal cases involving student nurses can be used for exploring the legal duties and responsibilities of the student, preceptor, and faculty. This topic always generates a number of questions from participants.

Preceptor Manual

Because it is not possible for all staff nurses to attend the workshop, developing a manual summarizing the workshop's essential information is important. This manual can also be given to those attending the workshop to use as a resource. It can be used when orienting any new preceptor on a one-to-one basis.

Future Directions for Preceptor Preparation

Considering health care agencies' limited resources, both material and human, alternative methods to prepare preceptors must be considered. Development of a web-based preceptor preparation course would allow potential preceptors to access the course at their convenience, decrease man power needed to teach the workshop, and be a resource available to preceptors at all times when working with students. Development of a preceptor course on CD or DVD could be individualized to each unit but also contain the general information usually presented in the workshop format. Previously videotaped guest speakers can be incorporated in either a web-based course, CD, or DVD. A mobile poster that could be moved from unit to unit could also be used to educate preceptors.

SUMMARY

This chapter has presented the process of developing and implementing an undergraduate preceptorship. The roles and responsibilities of the student, preceptor, and faculty were explored and linked to the success of an undergraduate preceptorship. The importance of maintaining clear, open lines of communication was a central theme throughout the chapter. A number of factors related to selecting appropriate preceptors and faculty were described. A model undergraduate preceptorship was used to highlight important policies and procedures. Finally, information necessary for preparing staff nurses for their preceptor role was described.

REFERENCES

American Association of Colleges of Nursing. (2004). *Thousands of students turned away from the nation's nursing schools despite sharp increase in enrollment.* Retrieved May 24, 2004, from http://www.aacn.nche.edu/Media/NewsReleases/enrl03.htm

Bain, L. (1996). Preceptorship: A review of the literature. *Journal of Advanced Nursing, 24,* 104–107.

Beeman, R. Y. (2001). New partnerships between education and practice: Precepting junior nursing students in the acute care setting. *Journal of Nursing Education, 40*(3), 132–134.

Chickerella, B. G., & Lutz, W. J. (1981). Professional nurturance: Preceptorships for undergraduate nursing students. *American Journal of Nursing, 81,* 107–109.

DeYoung, S. (2003). *Teaching strategies for nurse educators.* Upper Saddle River, NJ: Prentice Hall.

Gaberson, K. B., & Oermann, M. H. (1999). *Clinical teaching strategies in nursing.* New York: Springer Publishing.

Haas, B. K., Deardorff, K. U., Klotz, L., Baker, B., Coleman, J., & Dewitt, A. (2002). Creating a collaborative partnership between academia and service. *Journal of Nursing Education, 41*(12), 518–523.

Hseih, N. L., & Knowles, D. W. (1990). Instructor facilitation of the preceptorship relationship in nursing education. *Journal of Nursing Education, 29*(6), 262–268.

Lambert, V. A., & Lambert, C. E. (2001). Preceptorial experience. In A. J. Lowenstein & M. J. Bradshaw (Eds.), *Fuszard's innovative teaching strategies in nursing* (3rd ed., pp. 242–250). Gaithersburg, MD: Aspen.

Lengacher, C. A., & Tittle, M. B. (2000). Critical care in a baccalaureate program. *Nursing Connections, 13*(4), 69–76.

Manager's Forum. (2001). Preparing and compensating preceptors. *Journal of Emergency Nursing, 27*(3), 290–291.

Meng, A., & Conti, A. (1995). Preceptor development: An opportunity to stimulate critical thinking. *Journal of Nursing Staff Development, 11*(2), 71–76.

McCarty, M., & Higgins, A. (2003). Moving to an all graduate profession: Preparing preceptors for their role. *Nurse Education Today, 23,* 89–95.

Nordgren, J., Richardson, S. J., & Laurella, V. B. (1998). A collaborative preceptor model for clinical teaching of beginning nursing students. *Nurse Educator, 23*(3), 27–32.

Oermann, M. H. (1996). Research on teaching in the clinical setting. In K. R. Stevens (Ed.), *Review of research in nursing education: Volume VII* (pp. 91–126). New York: NLN Press.

Oulette, L. (1993). The relationship of a preceptor experience to the views about nursing as a profession of baccalaureate nursing students. *Nurse Education Today, 13,* 16–23.

Rittman, M. R., & Osburn, J. (1995). An interpretive analysis of precepting an unsafe student. *Journal of Nursing Education, 34*(5), 217–221.

Trevitt, C., Grealish, L., & Reaby, L. (2001). Students in transit: Using a self-directed preceptorship package to smooth the journey. *Journal of Nursing Education, 40*(5), 225–228.

CHAPTER 4

Precepting
in Acute Care

Janet Mackin and Carmen D. Schmidt

Т his chapter focuses on a preceptorship model for nurse orientees in an acute health care facility. The assumption is that the preceptorship is designed by a nurse educator who assumes responsibility for the program and for negotiating with orientees, preceptor, and nurse manager. Although the chapter is specific to this situation, many of the principles and practices discussed here would apply to other preceptorships as well.

This chapter provides preparatory information to

- design a preceptor training program,
- develop materials to support the preceptor role, and
- implement the preceptor role in the clinical setting.

PRINCIPLES INFLUENCING THE DESIGN OF A PRECEPTOR PROGRAM

Before getting into the specifics of designing a preceptor program, it is important to take an overview of the health care facility, the philosophy of the nursing department, the clinical and educational competence of the nursing staff, and the educational philosophy of the department. The goal is to develop a preceptor program that is well integrated within the structure of the health care facility.

An initial overall assessment will prevent adoption of a cookie-cutter model for a preceptor program.

As a starter, ask the following questions:

- **"What are the current mission, strategic plan, and specific goals of the health care facility?"** Not only should the mission and goals of the institution be implicitly and explicitly included in the content of the preceptor program, but they should be used as a guide to the program's design as well. In the rapidly changing health care field, the mission of an institution can change dramatically. For example, an institutional switch from a single-site facility to a networked organization should be reflected in the design of the preceptor program. Or, if improving patient satisfaction is high on the institution's list of goals, a customer relations component should be included in the functions of the preceptors and orientees. Case studies, orientee evaluation tools, and specific content may need to be adjusted to reflect these types of institutional changes.

- **"What are the philosophy, conceptual framework, and mission of the nursing department in the institution?"** The answer to this question should be consistent with the institutional mission and goals, but it should also provide some additional insights that will be important to a preceptor program. For example, preceptors should be more than familiar with the philosophy of the nursing department; they should be able to explain, apply, and, if necessary, defend it. This does not mean that they need to memorize the philosophy, but that they should feel its impact and implications in their practice. In addition, if the nursing department utilizes a specific conceptual framework, the preceptor program should be reviewed for consistency with each component of the framework.

- **"What is the level of the nursing staff's clinical competence?"** In some institutions, one has the luxury of working with a highly skilled, experienced nursing staff. Under these circumstances, preceptor selection will not present a problem and the development of the learners' educational skills will be easier. The preceptor program for this group can be of a high caliber and comprehensive. On the other hand, the staff may be a group of fledglings in a new area of practice who are having a difficult time finding their own way. Selecting the most prepared of these nurses for preceptor training may require an evaluation of the nurse's potential for precepting rather than demonstrated performance. More often, however, one selects preceptors from a mixed group of practitioners. In the design of a preceptor program for a diverse group, the match between learner and preceptor is important. One wants to build in an opportunity for more savvy preceptors to share their insights and experience with those learners who are a little shaky about a new role. Preprogram preparatory activities may help put preceptors and learners at more equal starting points.

• **"What is the educational philosophy of the nursing education department?"** In general, the most likely answer to this question is "an adult education philosophy." Years ago, the concepts of adult learning (Knowles, 1970) became a standard feature in nursing education. Since then, competency-based models and critical thinking approaches have gained support. Whatever the conceptual framework chosen, if "swallowed whole," one may find inconsistencies between what is said and what is done. For example, to espouse a critical thinking approach but to ignore or discourage questions is not "walking the walk." Nurse educators need to role model both clinical and educational standards for new staff members as well as nurses who are functioning as preceptors. It is wise for the nursing education staff to be on the alert for deviations from espoused beliefs and day-to-day practice. If nurse educators do not challenge themselves on their ability to put principles into practice, their preceptors will.

Taking the time to think through the implications of answers to the above questions will help to situate the preceptor program appropriately in the institution. A generic approach to designing a preceptor program will fail to meet the needs of the preceptors, orientees, and the institution.

PRECEPTOR SELECTION CRITERIA

As part of the design of the preceptor training program, prerequisites for preceptor selection should be developed and then shared with nurse managers. The nurse manager will need to be involved in identifying staff members eligible for the training program. Some suggested prerequisites include

TABLE 4.1 Criteria for Preceptor Selection

An ability to role model professional behavior
1. successful completion of all aspects of orientation to the assigned unit
2. performance evaluation that exceeds the minimum requirements
3. current proficiency in all items identified on the unit-specific skills monitor
4. current Basic Life Support/Advanced Life Support certification
5. mandatory educational requirements fulfilled

Demonstrated support of the philosophy of the nursing department
6. participation in at least one nursing committee, a hospital committee, or a unit-based project
7. willingness to assume additional responsibilities as necessary

An ability to communicate effectively
8. gives accurate, efficient, and effective shift reports
9. delivers clear, appropriate, and accurate patient education
10. communicates well with all members of the interdisciplinary team

A desire to precept new staff members
11. has completed the preceptor application/assessment form or volunteered for the Preceptor Training Program
12. has conducted informal staff education activities

- an ability to role model professional behavior,
- demonstrated support of the philosophy of the nursing department,
- an ability to communicate effectively, and
- a desire to precept new staff members.

Specific criteria for each of the prerequisites need to be defined (see Table 4.1).

During the Preceptor Training Program, the selection criteria should be reviewed with the preceptor candidates. This initial feedback will help reinforce the preceptor's commitment to the program and the new role. Preceptors should be made to feel special from the program's outset.

CONTENT OF THE PRECEPTOR TRAINING PROGRAM

Three broad content areas need to be addressed when designing a preceptor training program. First, preceptors need to be provided with a sound foundation in the principles of adult education. Secondly, they need to be given guidance in the clinical teaching and evaluation aspects of their new role. Specifically, this means that they will need to know the standards and tools that are used in guiding and evaluating a new nurse. Finally, preceptors need to be reassured that help is available after the program and be provided with ongoing support strategies.

FOUNDATION PRINCIPLES AND CONCEPTS

Characteristics of the Adult Learner

A review of adult learner characteristics (see chapter 2) should be included as part of the core content of the preceptor program. Frequently, preceptors have been exposed to adult education concepts and principles during their basic education and, it is hoped, during their orientation to the institution. However, at these times preceptors were on the receiving end of the educational process and were focusing on educational content, rather than educational strategies. As preceptors, they will need to utilize adult education strategies to enable the orientee to succeed. The ability to understand the adult learner will greatly assist in orientee assessment and appropriate assignment planning.

Roles and Responsibilities

Preceptors need to see the "big picture" of the orientation process and where they fit into it. Usually, preceptors are reassured to learn that there are four professionals involved in the orientation process: the orientee, the preceptor, the nurse manager, and the nurse educator. After learning that they are not on their own, preceptors are eager to know where their responsibilities begin and end. During the preceptor program, an outline of the specific responsibilities assigned to each role should be reviewed in order to provide the preceptor with a description of expected roles. The following are examples of responsibilities that might be assigned to each of the roles.

Orientee Responsibilities

- with the assistance of the preceptor and the nurse educator, identifies goals and objectives for orientation based on learning needs

- utilizes available resources to meet learning needs
- assumes increasing responsibility for patient care with preceptor guidance
- participates with the preceptor, nurse manager, and nurse educator in the appraisal process
- evaluates the orientation program, including the preceptor component

Preceptor Responsibilities

- attends the Preceptor Training Program
- with the orientee and nurse educator, identifies goals and objectives for orientation based upon learning needs
- serves as a bridge for the orientee's social integration into the unit
- plans the orientee's assignment, based upon the orientee's input and an objective assessment
- role models professional practice for the orientee
- acts as a clinical resource and support
- provides feedback to the orientee, the nurse manager, and the nurse educator
- identifies problems and refers them to the nurse manager and the nurse educator
- coordinates the orientee's clinical assignment with the orientation content
- utilizes orientation tools
- participates in the appraisal process with the orientee, the nurse manager, and the nurse educator
- evaluates the Preceptor Program

Nurse Manager Responsibilities

- selects a preceptor for each orientee
- schedules the preceptor's time and assignment to ensure availability for the orientee
- supports the preceptor and the orientee in problem identification
- provides feedback to the preceptor and the orientee

- participates in the appraisal process with the orientee, the preceptor, and the nurse educator
- evaluates the Preceptor Program

Nurse Educator Responsibilities

- provides the orientee with general orientation content
- assists the nurse manager in selecting a preceptor for each orientee
- assists the preceptor and the orientee in identifying the goals and objectives for the orientation
- role models professional practice for the preceptor
- provides preceptor training, guidance, support, and feedback
- assists the preceptor and the orientee in problem identification and provides additional instruction or clinical supervision when indicated
- participates in the appraisal process with the orientee, the preceptor, and the nurse manager
- evaluates the preceptor

Assessment and Socialization

Nurses are familiar with patient assessment. During the preceptor training program, preceptors need to learn how to refine their assessment skills for use with new staff nurses. The education program needs to emphasize the principles and process of assessment. Emphasizing the positive aspects of assessment helps to relieve preceptors of their fear of judging other nurses. Preceptors should be guided in how to conduct an initial assessment with an orientee and to ascertain the following:

- the orientee's educational background and past work experience,
- the orientee's self-assessment data, and
- the orientee's self-report of concerns or fears.

In addition, preceptors should be instructed in how to do an ongoing assessment of the orientee's abilities. To do this, the preceptor will need to understand the importance of providing a variety of meaningful clinical experiences and advance the difficulty and level of responsibility appropriately. During the program the preceptor should learn to appreciate the fact that assessment skills correlate closely with adult education concepts. Using case studies can help new preceptors understand the importance of assessing the orientee, observing the orientee's performance, and discussing clinical activities. The more preceptors understand their assessment responsibilities as they relate to the adult learner, the clearer will become the concept that orientation or learning is a shared responsibility.

The socializing role of the preceptor should also be stressed in the program. Research studies have shown that preceptors not only serve as an "on the spot resource" for clinical situations, but also facilitate the orientee's integration into the unit's social milieu. Kramer, who describes "reality shock" experienced by new graduates (1974) and Gardner (1992), who connects interpersonal conflict to job satisfaction, performance, and staff turnover, talk about the significance of support from experienced nurses in the acculturation of new nurses to their units. Winter-Collins and McDaniel's 2000 study notes that new graduate nurses need extra mentoring and nurturing to identify with the work setting and become part of the health care team. Ways to accomplish this should be covered in the Preceptor Training Program. The following can be presented as simple suggestions:

- introduce the orientee to unit personnel and other members of the health care team,
- review the unit's system for patient care delivery,
- provide information regarding roles and responsibilities of the members of the health care team, and
- involve the orientee in unit activities and routines.

Preceptors participating in the training program can be challenged to identify additional ways in which they can help to acculturate the new staff nurse.

Learning Styles

The Preceptor Training Program is an excellent opportunity to familiarize clinical experts with the concept of learning styles.

Sometimes clinical experts expect all learners to assimilate information in a fashion similar to their own. The rationale goes thus: "I learned to become a good nurse by (observing others/studying the theory/practicing/experimenting/etc.) and it worked for me. Therefore, it is the best way to learn for every new nurse." The logic derived from personal experience can be misleading and often inhibits the preceptor's ability to understand the learning styles of others.

At a minimum, the Preceptor Training Program should include a review of the basic learning styles. The work of Kolb (1993) is a useful model for understanding learning styles. Unfortunately, if presented as pure theory, the import and impact of this information may not be appreciated by preceptors. An experiential model for teaching learning styles may be more effective. The following exercise (Mulqueen, 1995) is an example of a participative method for presenting the teaching of learning styles. In this example, the Kolb Learning Style Inventory is used, but other learning assessment tools can be used in a similar fashion.

Exercise 1: Learning Styles

At the beginning of the program, all preceptors complete a learning style assessment. Scored assessments reveal each individual's learning style. At a later point in the program, participants are grouped at tables according to their learning styles. There is no need to tell participants why they are assigned to a particular group. Most frequently, there is a rather equal distribution of learning styles within a class. The group assignment is to create an object that represents the group. Colored paper, markers, old magazines, and any other interesting objects may be used by the group.

Educators who have done this exercise over and over again are amazed at the consistency of the results. If the Kolb Learning Styles Inventory is used, for example, the groups that prefer "Active Experimentation" and "Concrete Experience" are usually complaining that there are not enough supplies. They use up every minute feverishly building their object. The people whose learning styles fall into the categories of "Abstract Conceptualization" and "Reflective Observation" are usually slow to execute the project. These types of learners frequently need to clarify the rules and the purpose of the exercise and are somewhat embarrassed about their lack of activity. However, their thoughtful probing of the issue usually reveals some surprising insights.

At the end of the exercise, time is allocated to review each of the learning styles. This allows members from each of the groups to give examples of the group's learning style. For example, members of the "Abstract Conceptualization" group are likely to bring up the fact that they needed to have a theory of what their object would be before they could start construction. "Concrete Experience" group members may state that they felt better once they got their hands on the materials they would be using.

The facilitator of this session will need to lead the groups in further discussion of how this information can be used when they are precepting an orientee. Having discovered their own learning style preference and seeing that it is not the only way of learning, preceptors are more likely to be tolerant of orientees whose learning styles are different from their own. In addition, by providing a learning activity that allows for concrete experience, active experimentation, abstract conceptualization, and reflective observation, the Preceptor Training Program facilitator is able to model and reinforce the information regarding learning styles (Mulqueen, 1995).

Cultural Diversity

Preceptor candidates are usually familiar with some aspects of cultural diversity. Basic nursing school curricula normally include a component dealing with issues of cultural diversity as they pertain to patients. However, including information on cultural diversity in a preceptor program is also recommended. With the influx of large numbers of foreign nurses and the mobility of nurses within the United States, the probability is high that a preceptor will be asked to work with an orientee from a substantially different cultural, religious, or ethnic background. During the Preceptor Training Program, the topic of cultural diversity should be examined from a variety of viewpoints. Consider including some of the following approaches.

Cultural Stereotypes and How They Influence Our Expectation

Even those most critically aware of how cultural stereotyping influences behavior need a "booster shot" from time to time. For those less aware of their hidden assumptions regarding cultural differences, program content on diversity is an opportunity for them to explore their thoughts and feelings on the topic. For those with blatant prejudices, a cultural diversity program is essential either to change their opinions or to prevent them from inflicting their prejudices on orientees. Consider using prepackaged, professionally produced programs or developing an exercise activity. One effective class exercise is to form teams and have participants identify as many commonly held stereotypes as possible for different cultural groups. For example, one group would be assigned to list stereotypes associated with Hispanic Americans, another group would do the same for African Americans, and another group for Asian Americans. On completing the lists, the class as a whole could analyze how many of the stereotypes are negative. The group could also be prompted to examine how quickly and easily they were able to make the lists, which indicates how prevalent these prejudices are in society. Utilizing educators who are sensitive to cultural diversity issues is important to the success of this exercise. A team-teaching approach can work very well, especially if the team is culturally diverse.

Cultural Transition Processes and Issues

Preceptors need to have an awareness of some of the physical, emotional, educational, and social transitions required of foreign or newly relocated staff members. Although these nurses most likely have a theoretical awareness of the difficulty of making a transition, they may need assistance in gaining a sensitivity and true appreciation for just how difficult these transitions can be. Storytelling can be an excellent method for approaching these issues in the affective domain. Allowing preceptors to share their own experiences of transition with the group is one way in which participants can develop empathy for the nurse experiencing a cultural transition.

Cultural Differences Related to Learning Styles and Professional Practice

There are specific facts about the education and professional practice of nurses from different cultures that need to be shared with preceptors. For example, nurses from the Philippines have a baccalaureate degree as their basic entry into practice, and in their country they are assisted in the personal care of their patients by a variety of the patient's family members and friends. With this information, preceptors will be able to help Filipino nurses deal with the different support systems and responsibilities nurses have in the United States. The presence or lack of a college degree in nursing is important in the United States. Nurses from the Caribbean need to be prepared for this, as diploma schools still flourish in these countries. Nurses from Germany are accustomed to giving morning care at 3 or 4 A.M. and need to know that this is not the practice in the United States. The list could go on and on. To present pertinent information of this nature to the preceptor group, consider inviting staff members from a variety of cultural backgrounds to the training program. These "cultural representatives" can speak on their personal experiences of acclimating to American nursing. A question/answer session can also be an effective way for the preceptor group to learn from these individuals about cultural differences.

Problem-Solving Strategies

Whatever the time limitations of the Preceptor Training Program, discussing all the unusual and challenging situations that preceptors can face will be impossible. Some time must be saved for discussing problem-solving strategies. The preceptor group should be encouraged to identify as many problem-solving techniques as possible. Their lists should include suggestions such as the following:

* providing time for reflection and analysis before determining an approach to a problematic situation,
* defusing techniques,
* validating behavior and clarifying expectations,
* role modeling, and
* seeking expert assistance/guidance.

Critical Thinking Skills

The Preceptor Training Program should guide preceptors in methods that can support and develop the critical thinking abilities of the orientee. Research has shown that some preceptors are

hesitant about asking questions or challenging orientees' precon-
ceptions (Myrick, 2002). The Preceptor Training Program is an
excellent opportunity to guide preceptors into the type of dialogue
that will encourage reflection and critical analysis by the orientee.
In addition, the program provides nurse educators with a chance
to role model behaviors to stimulate critical thinking and establish
a relationship with preceptors that will continue beyond the program. The nurse educator becomes a mentor to preceptors, creating a chain of support for critical thinking within the institution.

Providing Feedback

Knowing how to provide feedback in a helpful, nonthreatening
fashion is one of the most important qualities of a successful preceptor. This ability enhances the orientee's trust of the preceptor and
the ability to really hear what the preceptor is saying. During the
Preceptor Training Program, techniques for providing constructive feedback should be reviewed and practiced. Table 4.2 identifies
some characteristics of helpful, nonthreatening feedback.

Clinical Teaching

Staff nurses are either selected or volunteer for the Preceptor
Training Program because they have demonstrated clinical expertise, the ability to role model professional nursing behavior, and
the desire to teach new nurses. Educators conducting the preceptor
training program must feel comfortable acknowledging the preceptors' competence. Nurse educators help preceptors to identify and
feel confidence in their strengths. As the program progresses,
educators should define clinical expertise in a way that does not
intimidate preceptors with the idea of being an expert. An important outcome of a Preceptor Training Program is that preceptors recognize both their present level of expertise and the
opportunity for further growth as professional nurses. Becoming
a preceptor is often the first step beyond the staff nurse role leading
to advanced practice roles such as clinical specialist, nurse educator,
and nurse manager.

The best preceptor training programs combine didactic information with an interactive or case-study process. Experienced
nurses in such a program will critically analyze real-life or simulated

TABLE 4.2   Characteristics of Positive Feedback

Focusing on the behaviors rather than the inferences: For example, "You finished all parts of the admission assessment except that the blood pressure was not recorded" is preferable to "Don't you know enough to take a patient's blood pressure when you admit him?"

Using descriptive rather than judgmental terms: For example, "Your hand was shaking when you gave the injection" is preferable to "You were a nervous wreck."

Discussing specific situations rather than abstractions: For example, "You seem to have had difficulty teaching Mrs. A. about her diabetic diet" is preferable to saying "You really have problems with patient teaching."

Sharing ideas rather than giving advice: "Have you considered" is a good opener for sharing ideas. In contrast, "Listen to me" narrows communication to a one-way street.

Exploring alternatives rather than providing solutions: Asking questions, such as, "Can you think of any other way that you might handle the situation?" can yield interesting results, whereas a statement such as, "There's only one thing you can do about it now" closes the door to creative thinking on the part of the orientee.

Limiting the amount of feedback at any one time: Even the most motivated orientee is limited in the amount of feedback that can be processed at one time. Giving too much, too soon is like asking the orientee to drink from a fire hose rather than a fountain of wisdom.

Making sure that feedback is given in a respectful, confidential manner: The center of the nurse's station is not a good location for giving feedback. Finding a quiet spot to discuss the orientee's progress demonstrates a caring, respectful concern for the new staff member.

Remembering that feedback is not a venting session for the preceptor: Even the best preceptors can become frustrated with their orientees; new preceptors need to be prepared to expect this. Preceptors need to identify venting techniques and support systems for themselves; otherwise, preceptors can inappropriately lash out at an orientee, which results in *two* very embarrassed nurses.

---

scenarios involving orientees, preceptors, patients, family members, and other unit staff. Discussion should focus on recognition and management of problem orientee behaviors as well as identifying preventive or corrective actions. Educators should review with preceptors the assessment tools used to evaluate baseline knowledge and to document ongoing development of new nurses' clinical skills. This review has a dual purpose: it reinforces the competence and ability of preceptors and helps preceptors recall all the clinical skills that they will be assessing in the orientees they precept. Preceptors should be competent in all the skills listed on the clinical skills checklist. If preceptors believe they have deficits in any of the competencies they will be validating in their orientees, educators should help them identify ways to update their skills.

Effective preceptors must be competent in the following areas:

- patient care skills,
- organizational skills,
- critical thinking or problem-solving skills, and
- communication skills with patients/families, and coworkers.

In order to plan assignments, the preceptor needs to be aware of the content of the orientation program for new nurses. For example, the orientee must successfully complete the intravenous therapy (IV) learning activities, including return demonstration of the IV pump, before being assigned to a patient receiving IV fluids. During the clinical portion of the orientation, the preceptor's responsibility is to provide progressive, challenging assignments. The goal is to increase the orientee's independence, while always protecting the patient's safety and comfort. At the same time, a preceptor should intervene to rescue an orientee who is in trouble. Finally, the preceptor must document clinical experiences in which the orientee has either assisted or observed.

Orientation Model and Tools

Orientation programs usually have two components: a didactic part (composed of classroom experiences, self-learning modules, or a combination of the two) and a clinical segment. Preceptors should be familiar with the most up-to-date version of all tools used throughout the orientation period: orientation calendars, schedules, assessment tools, plans, and resource materials. During the Preceptor Training Program the purpose and use of each orientation tool and its implication for the preceptor need to be spelled out in detail. The following are samples and descriptions of tools that should be reviewed with preceptors.

Clinical Skills Checklist

Although skills may vary from institution to institution and unit to unit, the design of the competency validation tool (skills checklist) need not vary (see Table 4.3). The skills checklist should have directions, a section for self-assessment, a rating scale, and a sign-off mechanism. A performance standard is also recommended to indicate the level of expertise the orientee is expected to achieve by the end of the orientation period. The preceptor should be aware that the orientee might not be able to demonstrate competency in all skills on the list, either because patient experience is not available during the orientation or because fully mastering the skill will require more time.

Scheduling

In an ideal orientation experience, the orientee should have all clinical days with the same preceptor. The nurse educator should consult in advance with the nurse manager about preceptor assignments in an effort to minimize the distress orientees frequently experience when working with multiple preceptors. Orientees can, of course, sometimes gain valuable insights when it is necessary to use more than one preceptor (e.g., different ways of organizing the tasks for the shift, different interpersonal styles, etc.).

Providing the preceptor with a calendar of the orientee's schedule will help the preceptor plan activities necessary to meet the learning needs of the orientee. Some institutions place the orientee on the same schedule as the preceptor, including weekends. Although nurse educator support is not usually available on weekends, the consistency of maintaining a link to the preceptor usually outweighs this drawback. If the orientee has been hired to work the evening or night shift, placement with a preceptor on the assigned shift is desirable. The orientee most commonly begins clinical orientation on the day shift. Transition to the assigned shift will then be dependent on the orientee's progress.

The greater the flexibility of the orientation program, the more complex the calendar can become. If all the didactic components of the orientation are scheduled at the same time every month, the schedule is straightforward. If the orientation is highly individualized and includes self-learning materials, classes, and off-unit clinical experiences (e.g., an observational experience in the operating room), coordinating the orientee's activities requires cooperation among the manager, preceptor, orientee, and educator.

TABLE 4.3 Sample of Competency Clinical Skills Checklist

Medical-Surgical RN Skills Checklist

Name: _____ Unit: _____

Purpose: This inventory of required nursing skills is to be completed by the end of your probation. You are responsible for having your preceptor or clinical specialist sign off on each skill after you demonstrate competency. Keep this document current and present it to the Nurse Manager for evaluation purposes. After probation, this document will become part of your personnel record.

Directions:
Read each competency and select a code from the following list that best describes your knowledge and/or experience. Put the code number you select in the column labeled "Self-Assessment."

Performance Code
1 = No experience
2 = Perform with assistance
3 = Perform under supervision
4 = Perform independently
N/A = Not applicable to unit or hospital site

Each time you demonstrate a skill, have the preceptor or clinical specialist or nurse manager initial and date a code number that best describes your skill level. You are expected to reach the performance standard for most of the competencies by the end of the probation period. Your nurse manager will review this checklist with you throughout the orientation and probationary period.

MEDICAL-SURGICAL NURSING SKILLS CHECKLIST

COMPETENCY	Self-Assessment Code #	Observer to initial & date under Code #	Performance Standard
		1 2 3 4	
I. Assessment:			
A. Measure patient's vital signs:			
1. TPR			4
2. Blood pressure			4
3. Neurological checks (orientation to time, place, person; response to directions and pain stimuli, pupillary reaction, extremity movement)			4

TABLE 4.3 *(continued)*

MEDICAL-SURGICAL NURSING SKILLS CHECKLIST

COMPETENCY	Self-Assessment Code #	Observer to initial & date under Code #				Performance Standard
		1	2	3	4	
4. Height						4
5. Weight						4
II. Planning:						
A. Write initial plan of care—nursing diagnosis/need/focus/discharge planning and patient teaching needs						4
B. Establish goal(s) with patient/family/SO						4
C. Write nursing interventions						4
III. Implementation:						
A. Maintain respiratory function:						
1. Administration of oxygen—set up, initiate and administer:						
a. Nasal cannula						4
b. Face mask						4
c. Venti mask						4
d. Nonrebreathing mask						4
e. Trach collar						4
f. T-piece						4
2. Incentive spirometer—demonstrate use of						4
3. Coughing and deep breathing—demonstrate and work with patient						4
4. Suctioning—lubricate catheter if applicable, insert, suction, and withdraw						

(continued)

TABLE 4.3 *(continued)*

MEDICAL-SURGICAL NURSING SKILLS CHECKLIST

COMPETENCY	Self-Assessment Code #	Observer to initial & date under Code #				Performance Standard
		1	2	3	4	
a. Nasotracheal						3
b. Oropharyngeal						3
c. Nasopharyngeal						3
5. Tracheotomy care— perform tube care, clean wound, change dressing, document						3
6. Closed chest drainage—observe for leaks, maintain, measure output, assess and document respiratory status, assess dressing						
a. Gravity						3
b. Suction						3
7. Pulse oximeter—set up, apply sensor, set alarms, reassure, interpret, record						3
8. Suction equipment— set up and maintain						
a. Portable suction						4
b. Wall suction						4
9. Respiratory assist devices—set up and maintain						
a. CPAP for sleep apnea						2
b. BIPAP						2

TABLE 4.3 *(continued)*

MEDICAL-SURGICAL NURSING SKILLS CHECKLIST

COMPETENCY	Self-Assessment Code #	Observer to initial & date under Code #				Performance Standard
		1	2	3	4	
10. Ventilator management—identify FIO$_2$, rate, TV mode. Respond, reset, and interpret alarms. Check humidification source and vent temperature. Empty excess water from tubing and administer nebulized medication						2
B. Maintain cardiovascular function:						
1. Code management:						
a. Verbalize emergency number to call						4
b. Initiate and administer BCLS						4
c. Bring code cart and EKG machine						4
d. Attach O$_2$ to Bag-Valve-Mask resuscitator						4
e. Prepare suction machine						4
f. Prepare code medications						4
2. Code cart and equipment maintenance—check cart, check O$_2$ tank, check suction and EKG machine						4

(continued)

TABLE 4.3   *(continued)*

MEDICAL-SURGICAL NURSING SKILLS CHECKLIST

COMPETENCY	Self-Assessment Code #	Observer to initial & date under Code #				Performance Standard
		1	2	3	4	
3. Blood products:						
a. Check, administer, and document blood product administration						3
b. Monitor patient during administration						3
c. State policy/procedure to use with transfusion reaction						3
C. Support and maintain nutritional requirements:						
1. TPN, PPN, Intralipids—administer and document						4
2. Tube feeding—check for placement, administer feedings, check and record residual						
a. Nasogastric						4
b. Gastrostomy						3
c. Jejunostomy						3
3. Intravenous therapy (peripheral, intermittent infusion devices)						
a. Verify order						4
b. Insert line/device and label dressing						4
c. Label bag and tubing						4
d. Calculate and regulate rate						4
e. Flush intermittent infusion device						4

TABLE 4.3 *(continued)*

MEDICAL-SURGICAL NURSING SKILLS CHECKLIST

COMPETENCY	Self-Assessment Code #	Observer to initial & date under Code #				Performance Standard
		1	2	3	4	
f. Assess and document site condition						4
4. Central line/Peripherally inserted central line catheter care						
a. Assess, change dressing, document site condition						4
b. Access central venous access catheter with subcutaneous reservoir						3
c. Flush/heparinize as per policy/procedure or as ordered by MD						3
D. Administer medications:						
1. Oral						4
2. Nasogastric						4
3. Subcutaneous						4
4. Intramuscular						4
5. Intravenous via peripheral line, intermittent infusion device, central line						4
6. Rectal						4
7. Vaginal						4
8. Ophthalmic						4
9. Otic						4
10. Topical						4
11. Patient Controlled Analgesia (PCA)						4
12. Nebulization						

(continued)

TABLE 4.3 *(continued)*

MEDICAL-SURGICAL NURSING SKILLS CHECKLIST

COMPETENCY	Self-Assessment Code #	Observer to initial & date under Code #				Performance Standard
		1	2	3	4	
13. Metered Dose Inhaler (MDI) with spacer						4
E. Care for patient with limited mobility:						
1. Pressure ulcer management—assess risk factors, document stage/observation, initiate and maintain skin care protocol						4
2. Range of motion exercises—initiate and maintain skin care protocol						4
3. Protective positioning and turning						4
4. Transfer to chair						4
5. Transfer to stretcher						4
6. Ambulation						
a. With assistance						4
b. Cane						3
c. Crutches						3
d. Walker						3
7. Care of patient with immobilizing device						
a. Cast						3
b. Traction						3
c. Sling						3
F. Maintain elimination function of GI and GU systems:						

TABLE 4.3   *(continued)*

MEDICAL-SURGICAL NURSING SKILLS CHECKLIST

COMPETENCY	Self-Assessment Code #	Observer to initial & date under Code #				Performance Standard
		1	2	3	4	
1. Care of the patient with naso-gastric tube—check for placement and pat-ency, maintain suc-tion, check bowel sounds, perform na-sal care, and docu-ment						4
2. Enemas						
a. Fleets						4
b. TWE						4
c. Retention						4
3. Ostomy care						
a. Skin care						4
b. Observation of stoma						4
c. Application of ap-pliance						4
d. Irrigation (with cone only), if ap-plies						3
4. Catheterization—insert, maintain, re-cord output, provide perineal care, re-move						
a. Indwelling						4
b. Straight						4
5. Suprapubic catheter care						3
6. External catheter (condom)						4
7. Peritoneal dialysis						
a. Initiate peritoneal dialysis						3

(continued)

TABLE 4.3 *(continued)*

MEDICAL-SURGICAL NURSING SKILLS CHECKLIST

COMPETENCY	Self-Assessment Code #				Observer to initial & date under Code #	Performance Standard
	1	2	3	4		
b. Add medications						3
c. Perform solution exchange						3
d. Obtain dialysate culture and cell count						3
e. Perform catheter and exit site care						3
f. Terminate peritoneal dialysis						3
G. Collect specimens:						
1. Stool for occult blood						4
2. Urine for urinalysis						4
3. Urine for culture and sensitivity						
a. Indwelling						4
b. Clean catch						4
4. 24-hour urine collection						4
5. Urine for S & A						4
6. Wound for C & S						4
7. Sputum for C & S						4
8. Sputum for AFB						4
9. Blood glucose monitoring						4
H. Implement principles of infection control:						
1. Handwashing						4
2. CDC isolation categories						4
3. Universal precautions						4
4. Sterile dressing changes						4

TABLE 4.3 *(continued)*

MEDICAL-SURGICAL NURSING SKILLS CHECKLIST

COMPETENCY	Self-Assessment Code #	Observer to initial & date under Code #				Performance Standard
		1	2	3	4	
5. Gowning, gloving, masking						4
6. Disposal of contaminated linen/trash						4
7. Handling of reusable equipment						4
8. Use of particulate respirators						4
I. Maintain patient, visitor, staff safety, environmental safety:						
1. Falls prevention—identify patient at risk, initiate and maintain patient safety alert protocol						4
2. Restraints—identify need, assess and provide comfort measures, renew order, document						4
3. Fall safe device—initiate, maintain, and monitor						4
J. Identify patient precautions (suicidal and nonsuicidal)—initiate, maintain, and document						4
K. Miscellaneous:						
1. Applies						
a. Abdominal binder						4

(continued)

TABLE 4.3 *(continued)*

MEDICAL-SURGICAL NURSING SKILLS CHECKLIST

COMPETENCY	Self-Assessment Code #	Observer to initial & date under Code #				Performance Standard
		1	2	3	4	
b. Elastic stockings, Ace bandages— observe peripheral circulation including color, sensation, capillary refill, skin temperature, peripheral pulse						4
2. Utilize equipment— set up, initiate, and monitor						
a. Hypo-/ hyperthermia blanket						4
b. Bedscale/chair scale						4
c. Electronic thermometer						4
f. Therapeutic bed						4
g. Infusion pump						4
h. Enteral feeding pump						4
i. Continuous Passive Motion (CPM) device						3
j. Hoyer lift						3
k. Sequential Compression device (SCD)						3
3. Maintain drains						
a. Jackson Pratt						3
b. Hemovac						3
4. Postmortem care						3
L. Document patient care:						
1. Admission nursing assessment						4

TABLE 4.3 *(continued)*

MEDICAL-SURGICAL NURSING SKILLS CHECKLIST

COMPETENCY	Self-Assessment Code #	Observer to initial & date under Code #				Performance Standard
		1	2	3	4	
2. Patient care plan/ MPC						4
3. Activity Flow Record						4
4. Nursing Treatment Kardex/MPC						4
5. Fluid Balance Record						4
6. Medication Administration Record (MAR)						4
7. Integrated Progress Notes						4
8. Preop checklist						4
9. Pre-/Postoperative Teaching Record						4
10. Informed consent						4
11. Transfer summary						4
12. Restraint flow sheet						4
13. Discharge nursing assessment						4
14. Patient discharge instructions						4
15. PCA Administration Record						4
16. Peritoneal dialysis flowsheet						3
17. Fingerstick accession quality control form						4
18. Pressure Ulcer Risk Assessment/Flow sheet						4
19. Patient Classification System, if applies						4

(continued)

TABLE 4.3 *(continued)*

IV. Other (unit specific)

Although the following are not strictly skills, you are expected to complete them and be independent upon completion of orientation:

COMPETENCY	Self-Assessment Code #	Observer to initial & date under Code #				Performance Standard
		1	2	3	4	
I. Admission (obtain report, prepare patient area, perform assessment, complete database, transcribe MD orders, write care plan and Kardex/MPC)						4
II. Intershift Report (give systematic assessment, identify needs, problems, and interdisciplinary intervention, administer care						4
III. Transfer (accept and send patients, write and give verbal report)						4
IV. Discharge (confirm discharge arrangements, complete discharge teaching, complete discharge summary and discharge instructions)						4
V. Patient Teaching (identify learning needs, provide and document teaching)						3
VI. Time Management (organize and prioritize patient care assignment, delegate appropriately)						3

TABLE 4.3 *(continued)*

COMPETENCY	Self-Assessment Code #	Observer to initial & date under Code #				Performance Standard
		1	2	3	4	
VII. Charge Nurse						
1. Assess patients' needs and skills levels of staff						3
2. Write and communicate staff's patient assignment, delegated tasks, scheduled meetings, and inservice classes						3
3. Assess and follow up Unit Secretary's performance of clerical and receptionist responsibilities						3
4. Orient floats to unit routine						4
5. Inform nursing office of unit staffing issues						3
6. Obtain periodic update of patient care needs/unit management issues from nursing staff. Communicate/facilitate communication of patient care/unit management issues to appropriate physician and designated nursing supervisor (Manager, Director)						3

Initials / Signatures / Title

_____ _____ _____

_____ _____ _____

_____ _____ _____

Orientation Clinical Summary:

_____

_____

_____

_____

(continued)

TABLE 4.3 *(continued)*

Signatures:

Nurse Educator: _____ Date: _____

Nurse Manager: _____ Date: _____

Preceptor: _____ Date: _____

Orientee: _____ Date: _____

The overall length of the actual orientation can also vary according to the assigned clinical area and/or the experience level of the new nurse. For example, an experienced medical-surgical nurse hired for a position in a Critical Care unit could be expected to pass an additional, comprehensive critical care education course, as well as the clinical orientation, to successfully complete orientation. Orientation to specialty units may be several months in duration. It may not be possible, in this situation, for the nurse manager to maintain the same preceptor assignment for the duration of the orientation.

Orientation Plans

Orientation plans are weekly guidelines used to help preceptors design the orientee's clinical experiences so that the orientee can achieve competence by the end of the orientation period. A 6-week medical-surgical orientation plan is provided as a sample in Table 4.4. The purpose of this plan is to provide the preceptor and the orientee with a framework for gradually advancing the number of assigned patients and the complexity of the skills to be mastered. Although all orientations should be competency based, these guidelines are based on the length of time and chronological order in which activities progress for an "average" orientee. Therefore, this sample plan should be considered a starting point and must be individualized, taking into account the experience of the nurse. It is designed to work in conjunction with the unit-specific clinical skills checklist, as presented above in Table 4.3.

Resource Materials

Orientees will get maximum benefit from the orientation if the preceptor is able to refer them to appropriate learning resources.

TABLE 4.4 Medical-Surgical Six-Week Orientation Plan and Competency/Skill Checklist

NAME: _____ UNIT: _____ DATE: _____

Purpose: To be used as a **guide** for the new RN as an introduction to the policies, procedures and role expectations of a Registered Professional Nurse in Medical-Surgical Nursing. This plan is to be used in conjunction with the following Self-Learning Modules (SLM)/checklists: Medication administration; 12 lead EKG; IV insertion; phlebotomy; CVAD, and any other unit specific checklist(s). Competency/skill to be validated on the appropriate checklist by preceptor and/or CNS and/or NM. **Each competency/skill must be performed successfully three (3) times in order for the RN to be checked off as competent.**

WEEK ONE: Week one is spent in the Division of Nursing Education completing the required classroom activities and covers one day of general human resources orientation, 6 days of general nursing orientation classes, and includes Monday and Tuesday of Week 2. The general nursing orientation combines self-learning modules (SLM), lectures, demonstrations, and skill labs with return demonstration by the orientee of hospitalwide nursing skills, including venipuncture, intravenous therapy, EKG, fingerstick blood glucose measurement, and patient controlled analgesia.

WEEK TWO: Week 2 begins the clinical segment of the nurse's orientation. Week 2 is the Wednesday, Thursday, and Friday immediately following completion of Nursing Orientation classroom activities.

COMPETENCY/SKILL	LEARNING RESOURCES/ ACTIVITIES	PRECEPTOR INITIALS/DATE

(Note: the opportunity to perform skills marked below with an asterisk * may not be available during week 2.)
 	
1. Complete scavenger hunt (Table 4.5) (to be done day 1 on the unit)
 	
   • Introduction to unit staff/preceptor (to be done day 1 on the unit)
   • Review dress code policy
	Scavenger hunt checklist
	Dress code: Human Resources Policy
	Code Cart: Code Cart Reference Manual
	Defibrillator: Procedures
	CPR Educational Requirements	

(continued)

TABLE 4.4   *(continued)*

COMPETENCY/SKILL	LEARNING RESOURCES/ ACTIVITIES	PRECEPTOR INITIALS/DATE
• Review Medical Record (MR)/chart; begin to become familiar with forms • Introduction to schedule; sign-in/swipe-in process • Introduction to paging system/key telephone #'s • Begin to review and/or check code cart/defibrillator (weekly check as per unit schedule—may not be able to do until week 3) • Attend multidisciplinary patient care rounds • Perform 12 lead EKG* • Insertion of Intravenous line* • Perform phlebotomy/venipuncture*	**Multidisciplinary Patient Care Rounds:** Refer to "Care Management" SLM distributed/ completed during orientation classes **12 lead EKG:** SLM; Procedure **IV insertion:** SLM; Procedure **Phlebotomy/venipuncture:** SLM; Procedures	
• Unit specific competencies/ self-learning packets/checklists, etc: • _____ • _____	**Unit specific competencies:** • _____ • _____	
2. **Begin to** develop, provide and document plan of care for _____ # of patients (recommend minimum of 3–4) based on patient diagnosis, treatments, medications, psychosocial status, etc. To include collaboration with multidisciplinary team, interaction with family, referrals, etc. **Note:** Preceptor and orientee are to have joint assignment of patients with orientee having total responsibility (**EXCEPT** for medication administration) for number of patients indicated above.	**Patient Plan of Care (Nursing Care Plan):** Refer to "Care Management" SLM distributed/completed during orientation classes **Patient Care Assignments:** Policy **Patient Bill of Rights:** Policy **Vital signs:** Policy **Weights/Heights:** Policy **Intake and Output:** Procedure **Allergies:** Policy **Food and Drug Interaction:** Policy	

TABLE 4.4   *(continued)*

COMPETENCY/SKILL	LEARNING RESOURCES/ ACTIVITIES	PRECEPTOR INITIALS/DATE
(**The Experienced RN** is expected to be capable of caring for larger number of patients than the **inexperienced RN or new graduate**.) Each week, the number of patients cared for by the orientee should increase. The goal is for the orientee to have total responsibility for a complete patient assignment with preceptor as resource by week 6.	**Assessment/Reassessment:** Policy **Visitors:** Policy **Discharge of a Patient:** Refer to "Care Management" SLM distributed/completed during orientation classes; Meet with Case Manager assigned to your unit.	

3. **If available**, initiate and complete one admission assessment, including physical assessment, under the supervision of preceptor (including assessment of breath sounds, bowel sounds, neurological and neurovascular status, peripheral pulses, etc.).

4. **If available**, initiate and complete one discharge summary under supervision of preceptor.

5. Weekly meeting with NM and preceptor (and CNS if available). Bring this weekly planner as well as any completed checklists to every weekly meeting.

Weekly meeting comments, action plan, etc. To be signed/dated by orientee, NM, and preceptor. Use back of paper if more space is needed:

(continued)

WEEK THREE

COMPETENCY/SKILL	LEARNING RESOURCES/ ACTIVITIES	PRECEPTOR INITIALS/DATE
1. Continue to perform competencies/skills identified in week 2.	**Medication Administration:** Policies and Procedures	
2. Continue to develop, provide and document plan of care for _____ # of patients (recommend minimum of 4–6) **with the addition of medication administration.**	**Blood Glucose Monitors:** Policy, Procedure **Oxygen administration:** Refer to "Respiratory Care" SLM distributed/completed during orientation classes; Procedures	
3. PBDS review with Nursing Education Manager	**Bag/Valve/Mask:** Refer to "Respiratory Care" SLM distributed/completed during orientation classes; Procedure	
4. **Begin to** give and accept verbal patient report: • Shift change • Postop • Postprocedure • Emergency Department • Unit-to-unit transfer • Interinstitutional	**Nebulizer Treatments:** Refer to "Respiratory Care" SLM distributed/completed during orientation classes; Procedure **Suctioning:** Procedures	

5. **Begin to** demonstrate proper use and required documentation of equipment frequently used in patient care:
• Manual and electronic BP machines
• Blood glucose monitor
• Infusion pumps
• Intravenous solutions/tubing
• Oxygen administration via:
   • nasal cannula
   • face mask (various concentrations)
   • rebreather mask
   • tracheostomy (collar) mask
   • bag-valve-mask
   • Suction equipment
   • Incentive spirometer
   • Use of pulse oximeter		

TABLE 4.4 *(continued)*

COMPETENCY/SKILL	LEARNING RESOURCES/ ACTIVITIES	PRECEPTOR INITIALS/DATE
6. Weekly meeting with NM and preceptor (and CNS if available)		
7. Unit specific competencies/self-learning packets/checklists, etc: • _____ • _____	**Unit specific competencies:** • _____ • _____	
8. **Begin to** become familiar with the following specific chart forms and/or policies/procedures: • Departmental and Institutional chain of command for reporting/support • Physician chain of command for reporting/support • Cardiac Arrest Code, disaster plan; fire safety (RACE—Rescue, Alarm, Contain, Extinguish) • Medication administration • Narcotics and controlled substances • Patient Notification Record (PNR) • Occurrence (Incident) reporting • Suicide precautions • Restraints: physical and chemical • Weekly skin risk assessment form • Pressure ulcer prevention and treatment • Standard Nursing Care Plans/individualization of • Interdisciplinary Patient /Family Education Record • Neurological assessment • Pain assessment/management: acute and chronic	**Patient/Family Education:** Refer to "Patient Teaching" SLM distributed/completed during orientation classes; Policies **Patient Plan of Care (Nursing Care Plan):** Refer to "Care Management" SLM distributed/completed during orientation classes; Policy **Medication Administration:** **Incentive Spirometer:** Procedure **Falls Prevention/Patient Falls:** Policies **Occurrence Reporting:** Policy **Skin Risk Assessment and Pressure Ulcer:** Refer to "Skin Risk Assessment Record & Pressure Ulcer Flow Sheet" SLM distributed/completed during orientation classes; Policy **Restraints:** Policy **Neurological Assessment:** See "Nursing Neurological Assessment" **Pain Assessment/Management:** Policy **Approved Abbreviations:** See list of Approved Abbreviations kept on each nursing unit	

(continued)

TABLE 4.4 *(continued)*

COMPETENCY/SKILL	LEARNING RESOURCES/ ACTIVITIES	PRECEPTOR INITIALS/DATE
• Pressure ulcer prevention and treatment; weekly tracking form • Falls risk assessment and prevention • Approved abbreviations		

Weekly meeting comments, action plan, etc. To be signed/dated by orientee, NM and preceptor:

WEEK FOUR

COMPETENCY/SKILL	LEARNING RESOURCES/ ACTIVITIES	PRECEPTOR INITIALS/DATE
1. Continue to develop, provide and document plan of care for _____ # of patients (recommend minimum of 6–8) including medication administration.		
2. Introduction to PYXIS and obtain personal PYXIS # from pharmacy (successful medication administration required).		
3. Perform shift change narcotics and controlled substances count (successful medication administration required).		
4. Weekly meeting with NM and preceptor (and CNS if available).		
5. Register for PRI (Peer Review Instrument) class.		

TABLE 4.4 *(continued)*

COMPETENCY/SKILL	LEARNING RESOURCES/ ACTIVITIES	PRECEPTOR INITIALS/DATE
6. Continue to perform competencies/skills identified in weeks 1 and 2 and begin to demonstrate competency in the following skills.		

Note: These competencies/skills should be performed as they present themselves on the unit. You may NOT have the opportunity to demonstrate competency in all skills during orientation AND not all skills may be applicable to your unit:

- Administration of blood and blood products
- Care of the patient with a Patient Controlled Analgesia (PCA) Pump:

  - Intravenous administration
  - Epidural administration
  - Subcutaneous administration

- Care of the patient with a Central Venous Access Device (CVAD):

  - Peripherally inserted Central Catheter (PICC)
  - Implanted port/use of Huber needle
  - Triple lumen catheter

- Urinary catheterization:

  - male
  - female

- Administration of total parenteral nutrition (TPN)

(continued)

TABLE 4.4   *(continued)*

COMPETENCY/SKILL	LEARNING RESOURCES/ ACTIVITIES	PRECEPTOR INITIALS/DATE

• Administration of lipids
• Enteral feedings including:
  • Nasogastric feeding tube (N-G tube)
  • Percutaneous Endoscopic Gastrostomy (PEG) tube
  • Gastrostomy tube (G-tube)
 	
• Care of the patient with an ostomy
• Care of the patient with a tracheostomy
• Care of the patient with a chest tube		

7. **Begin to** become familiar with the following specific chart forms and/or policies:

- Blood and blood products
- Alert values (critical lab values)
- Change in patient's condition
- Crisis resolution management
- Patient complaints
- Central venous access devices
- Enteral feedings
- Gastrostomy tube/PEG/Naso-gastric tube, etc.
- Ostomy care
- Patient Controlled Analgesia (PCA)
- Specimen collection
- Blood cultures
- Sequential compression devices (SCDs)
- Wound care
- Dressing changes

TABLE 4.4   *(continued)*

COMPETENCY/SKILL	LEARNING RESOURCES/ ACTIVITIES	PRECEPTOR INITIALS/DATE

• Hypothermia blankets
• Specialty beds/overlays: indications for, approval and ordering of
• Discharge Planning
  • Patient Review Instrument (PRI)
  • Assessment for Home Care Services (M11Q)
• Food-drug interactions guideline		

8. Unit specific competencies/self-learning packets/checklists, etc:
  • _____
  • _____
  • _____		

Weekly meeting comments, action plan, etc. To be signed/dated by orientee, NM, and preceptor. Use back of paper if more space is needed:

WEEK FIVE

COMPETENCY/SKILL	LEARNING RESOURCES/ ACTIVITIES	PRECEPTOR INITIALS/DATE
1. Continue to develop, provide and document plan of care for _____ # of patients (recommend 7–8), including medication administration.	**Patient Report:** Refer to "Care Management" SLM distributed/completed during orientation classes	

(continued)

TABLE 4.4   *(continued)*

COMPETENCY/SKILL	LEARNING RESOURCES/ ACTIVITIES	PRECEPTOR INITIALS/DATE
2. Continue to perform competencies/skills identified in weeks 2–4 and **demonstrate competency in the following** (Must perform successfully 3 times in order to be considered competent. If unable to perform 3 times due to lack of opportunity on your unit, please notify your NM and/or CNS and arrangements will be made to give you the opportunity to perform these skills in another area/unit.):		

- Independent completion of admission assessment/physical assessment, including assessment of breath sounds, bowel sounds, neurological status, etc.
- Independent completion of discharge summary including patient /family education, referrals, etc.
- Ability to give and accept verbal patient report:
  - Shift change
  - Postop
  - Postprocedure
  - Emergency Department
  - Unit-to-unit transfer
  - Interinstitutional

- Perform 12 lead EKG
- Insertion of intravenous line
- Perform phlebotomy/venipuncture
- Use of blood glucose monitor
- Use of Infusion pumps
- Use of paging system

TABLE 4.4 *(continued)*

COMPETENCY/SKILL	LEARNING RESOURCES/ ACTIVITIES	PRECEPTOR INITIALS/DATE

• Oxygen administration via:
  • nasal cannula
  • face mask (various concentrations)
  • rebreather mask
  • tracheostomy (collar) mask
  • bag-valve-mask
 	
• Set-up and use of suction equipment		

3. Unit specific competencies/self-learning packets/checklists, etc: • _____ • _____ • _____ • _____	**Unit specific competencies:** • _____ • _____ • _____ • _____	
4. Demonstrate competency in the following communication and critical thinking areas: • Demonstrate an understanding of the departmental and institutional chain of command • Demonstrate an understanding of the physician chain of command for reporting/support • Demonstrate an understanding of the various disciplines involved in patient care • Know how/when/whom to contact for reporting/support • Ability to prioritize the needs of the patients and the unit • Ability to clarify unclear situations as needed	**Critical Thinking:** Refer to "Delegation Decisions for the Registered Nurse" distributed/ completed during orientation classes;	

(continued)

TABLE 4.4 *(continued)*

COMPETENCY/SKILL	LEARNING RESOURCES/ ACTIVITIES	PRECEPTOR INITIALS/DATE
• Ability to respond quickly and appropriately in the event of unanticipated/ untoward situations • Ability to justify actions in a clear, concise manner		

Weekly meeting comments, action plan, etc. To be signed/dated by orientee, NM, and preceptor.

WEEK SIX

COMPETENCY/SKILL	LEARNING RESOURCES/ ACTIVITIES	PRECEPTOR INITIALS/DATE
1. Continue to perform competencies/skills identified in weeks 2–5.		
2. Continue to develop, provide and document plan of care for _____ # of patients (recommend 8) including medication administration. **Successful completion of orientation requires independent care of full patient assignment utilizing preceptor as resource only.**		
3. Weekly meeting with NM and preceptor (and CNS if available) and review of orientation/probation status.		

TABLE 4.4   *(continued)*

COMPETENCY/SKILL	LEARNING RESOURCES/ ACTIVITIES	PRECEPTOR INITIALS/DATE
4. **Nurses hired for evening and night shifts** will begin shift assignment and will continue to work with preceptor during weeks 6–8, if not sooner. At completion of week 8, there will be a review of orientation/ probation status with NM/preceptor and CNS if available.		

Weekly meeting comments, action plan, etc. To be signed/dated by orientee, NM, and preceptor. Use back of paper if more space is needed.

The Preceptor Training Program content should include a comprehensive review of available resource materials on site, such as the policy and procedure manuals on the patient care unit, textbooks and professional library materials, computer reference material, videocassette and CD education programs, and patient education materials. The Nursing Education Department may also have additional institution or specialty-specific learning packages or other materials to enrich the orientee's learning experience.

Program Format for Preceptor Training

The format of a Preceptor Training Program will depend on the amount of time allocated for training. Content could be covered in a half day or reviewed in detail with experiential exercises over a two-day period. A cost–benefit analysis should be used to justify the amount of time spent in training preceptors according to the benefits accrued as a direct result of the program.

Frequently, the most convenient, cost-effective, and educationally feasible vehicle for preceptor training is a one-day workshop. The program can be designed with interactive didactic presentations in the morning followed in the afternoon by presentation of case studies, exercises, questions and answers, and group problem solving. Prior to the program, preceptors should receive selected readings to review in preparation for the course. This precourse assignment assures that all participants have a minimum baseline of information.

The role of the Preceptor Training Program faculty is to review, reinforce, and clarify learning. Using real-life case studies as starting points (ideally contributed by preceptors from within the institution) faculty can help preceptors identify the principles that should guide their practice as preceptors. Rather than using a lecture format, the class should be arranged as a discussion or seminar. As a method of evaluation, a workshop element can be incorporated at the end of the program.

In the workshop, preceptors can be divided into groups and presented with orientation training scenarios. Using concepts learned during the program, the preceptor groups attempt to "solve" these scenarios. At the end of the workshop, each preceptor group presents its solution to the class. This format provides faculty with feedback about how well preceptors understand the principles of adult education and their responsibilities as preceptors. This approach also models a collaborative problem-solving technique that can be used in the clinical setting.

Another approach is to use role playing to dramatize the scenarios in the workshop. If the group is hesitant to engage in role playing, an alternative is to use videotaped role plays done either by the faculty or former preceptors. Participants can then analyze the role play and suggest or demonstrate alternative outcomes.

For institutions where preceptor enrollment is small and/or instructor resources are limited, the content of the Preceptor Training Program can be put into independent study format using e-learning or video programs, written reference materials, and self-assessment tools. Although this model is not preferred, it does adequately provide preceptors with a basic conception of their role, and its lack of group interaction is partly offset by the timeliness with which preceptor education can be provided. This means that the staff member does not have to wait several months for the next scheduled Preceptor Training Program, as self-instruction

TABLE 4.5 Medical-Surgical Scavenger Hunt Checklist

Name: _____ Unit: _____ Date: _____

Purpose: To assist new staff RNs to become familiar with the

- location of equipment, forms, supplies, and rooms on their assigned nursing unit.
- identities and roles of unit and non unit-based staff members with whom they will be working.

Directions: Place a check on the line when you have located the area or item on your unit. Submit the completed list to your Nurse Manager.

	Date Completed	NM/preceptor initials
Identifies unit staff members and responsibilities:		
• Nurse Manager _____	_____	_____
• Preceptor _____	_____	_____
• Case Manager _____	_____	_____
• Social Worker _____	_____	_____
• Patient Care Associates	_____	_____
• Unit Support Associates	_____	_____
• Housekeeping staff	_____	_____
Identifies non-unit based staff members and responsibilities:		
• Nurse Education Manager _____	_____	_____
• Clinical Nurse Specialist _____	_____	_____
• Nutritionist	_____	_____

(continued)

TABLE 4.5 *(continued)*

	Date Completed	NM/preceptor initials
• Dietician	————	————
• Pharmacist	————	————
• Attending Physician(s)	————	————
• Fellow(s)	————	————
• Residents	————	————
• Interns	————	————
• Physician's Assistant	————	————
• Nurse Practitioner	————	————
• Physical Therapist	————	————
• Occupational Therapist	————	————
• Speech Therapist	————	————
• Hospital Transporter	————	————
• Chaplain	————	————
• Patient Representative	————	————
• Other —————————	————	————

States location of:

• Nurses station	————	————
• Medication room	————	————
• Pantry/nourishment area	————	————
• Clean utility room	————	————
• Soiled utility room	————	————

TABLE 4.5 *(continued)*

	Date Completed	NM/preceptor initials
• Linen storage area	————	————
• Linen chute	————	————
• Bathtubs/showers	————	————
• Store room	————	————
• Wheelchair/stretcher storage	————	————
• Oxygen shut-off valve	————	————
• Oxygen/suction outlets	————	————
• Oxygen therapy supplies and suction equipment	————	————
• Intravenous and PCA pump storage area	————	————
• Policy and procedure manuals:		
Nursing	————	————
Human Resources	————	————
Administrative	————	————
• Patient education manual/resources	————	————
• Nursing Care Plans	————	————
• Frequently used chart forms, requisition slips, etc.	————	————
• Admission book	————	————
• Assignment sheet	————	————
• Supply closet and supplies location	————	————
• Fire alarms/extinguishers	————	————
• Conference room	————	————

(continued)

TABLE 4.5 *(continued)*

	Date Completed	NM/preceptor initials
• Locker room	____	____
• Other _____	____	____
• Other _____	____	____
• Other _____	____	____
• Other _____	____	____

_____

Employee signature

can occur at any time. If a self-instructional model is offered for preceptor training, either alone or as an adjunct to the group format, it can be supplemented with shorter, 2-hour workshops in which preceptors who have completed the self-instructional training can come together to discuss questions, problems, or concerns they are experiencing in their role as preceptors. This workshop would provide not only reinforcement and clarification of the role of the preceptor, but also group support that may have been missed by the preceptors in their initial training.

Preceptor Program Supports

Ideally, orientation is seen as a responsibility of all employees, not just the members of the education department. With the participation of peers, orientation becomes more than just a classroom exercise. Peer participation can transform orientation into a dynamic, meaningful learning experience. To support peer participation in orientation, job descriptions should be written to include the responsibility each staff member has in orienting a new member. At a minimum, a staff member should be able to assist in some way in the transition that takes the orientee from a neophyte to a colleague who can pull his/her own weight. Preceptors take this minimum expectation one step further. After receiving training, they are capable of providing a professional clinical orientation for the new nurse.

Internal motivating factors, usually the desire and satisfaction related to teaching, contribute greatly to the staff person's willingness to precept a new nurse. However, external motivators and rewards can make the role much more appealing.

Any one or a combination of the following strategies can be used to communicate to preceptors that the institution recognizes and acknowledges their commitment by

- offering continuing education credits for attending the Preceptor Training Program,
- presenting preceptors with a certificate and a pin,
- providing a salary differential for precepting,
- publishing preceptors' names and pictures in the hospital newsletter, and/or
- sending preceptors a letter of recognition from nursing leadership.

Recognition of preceptors should not be considered a "one-shot deal," as the preceptor role is one that requires daily commitment and can sometimes seem like a thankless task. A bad experience with one orientee can leave a preceptor dejected and erase any memories of the pluses originally associated with the role. Preceptors should be prepared for these bad times in their initial training. Such problems as mismatches between orientee and preceptor, orientee termination due to performance problems, or a variety of other pressures involved in being a preceptor should be discussed in the training program.

Ongoing support and recognition can help to alleviate preceptor burnout. These supports could include:

- a professional journal subscription,
- an annual Preceptor Recognition Reception,
- the opportunity to participate in additional continuing education activities,
- instructor feedback on preceptor skills,

- nurse manager feedback on preceptor involvement, and
- orientee evaluation of preceptor's role in orientation.

Supports like the ones listed above indicate to the preceptor that the institution is willing to support ongoing development in the preceptor role.

THE PRECEPTOR ROLE IN ACTION

Assignment Planning for the Orientee

There are three components involved in planning a clinical assignment for the orientee:

1. reviewing the orientee's self-assessment form,
2. providing observational experiences for the orientee, and
3. planning the patient-care assignment.

The first or fundamental component of planning the orientee's clinical assignment is the preceptor's *review of the orientee's self-assessment*. Before the first clinical experience, the orientee usually completes some version of an assessment tool to be shared with the preceptor. The preceptor reviews this tool, taking into consideration the orientee's educational background and past work experience. The assessment tool provides the preceptor with a concrete starting point related to the orientee's technical skills when selecting patient-care assignments.

The second component of assignment planning involves *providing observational experiences* for the orientee. Depending on the orientee's past experience, time devoted to observational experiences will vary. Observational experiences include activities such as shadowing the preceptor for the purpose of observing unit routines, patient-care activities, time management, and priority setting. An experienced nurse is usually ready for a modified independent patient-care assignment after one day of observing the preceptor. However, a new graduate might need additional observational time due to the sensory overload of a typical orientation.

The third component of assignment planning is the actual *patient-care assignment*. The orientee's patient assignment is made by the preceptor, if possible, with input from the orientee. This collaborative approach works well, not only at the beginning of orientation, but long after, when preceptor and orientee are true peers. In addition to using the skills monitor data to determine the assignment, the preceptor is encouraged to take into consideration the orientee's comfort level during the observational experience. If, for example, the orientee demonstrated extreme nervousness when talking with patients or staff members, the preceptor should start with an easier patient-care assignment, graduating the acuity of patients with increasing orientee confidence. The preceptor might initially choose to share his/her assignment with the inexperienced orientee. The two would work together in a "buddy system" and the preceptor would delegate aspects of patient care to the orientee. The preceptor would be right beside the inexperienced orientee as an "on the spot" resource and support. On the other hand, an experienced nurse whose questions and comments during the observational experience indicate a high level of knowledge and confidence might work independently from the start, using the preceptor as a resource.

Even with the best of planning, relevant patient-care experiences may be difficult to provide. A specific patient-care experience may not be available within the preceptor's assignment or in the clinical setting. Even if it involves shifting to a different location, arrangements should be made for the orientee to be assigned to a patient who provides a learning opportunity, ideally with the preceptor also covering the patient. This is preferable to the orientee being split between two preceptors. It is important for the preceptor to be committed to providing the orientee with as many experiences as feasible during the dedicated time of orientation when support and guidance are readily available.

When a relevant patient-care experience is not available in the clinical setting during orientation, other options are available. For example, the orientation period could be extended or a plan could be made to provide the experience after the orientation period. In the latter situation the orientee and the nurse manager need to mutually agree to seek out the experience when the opportunity presents itself.

Evaluating the Orientee

From the onset of orientation, the orientee shares responsibility for assessing learning needs, identifying and utilizing resources, and requesting specific patient-care assignments that validate his/ her competence. The preceptor, nurse educator, and nurse manager should respect the orientee's input and make tools, guidelines, and resources available to enable the orientee to succeed.

At the conclusion of orientation, the orientee should complete a summative self-evaluation. This could be the self-assessment tool used at the start of the orientation or could be the performance evaluation tool based on the job description. This summative evaluation is an opportunity for the orientee to note progress, problems, or concerns prior to assuming full staff responsibility. If the orientation has been successful, this self-evaluation is usually a satisfying experience for the orientee. If the orientation was problematic, the final self-evaluation is an opportunity for the orientee to identify specific weaknesses and discuss them with the nurse manager.

For some orientees self-evaluation is an intimidating and difficult process; however, it is an important skill that nurses will use on an ongoing basis during their careers. If care was taken during the initial self-assessment to make it a positive, nonthreatening situation, the summative self-assessment will be less intimidating. Orientees will have little temptation to give a falsely high or low rating of their skills if a nonpunitive approach is taken to skills assessment throughout orientation.

The orientee's self-assessment provides the starting point for the collaborative evaluation completed by the nurse manager, preceptor, and nursing instructor. Throughout the orientation the preceptor communicates with the nurse manager and nurse educator, providing updates on the orientee's progress. These update sessions should be conducted on a regularly scheduled basis, or as daily informal "on-the-go" communications. Based on these updates, orientation plans can be revised and made more responsive to the needs of the orientee.

Final Written Evaluation

The final assessment of the orientee, completed by the nurse manager, preceptor, and nurse educator, should reflect the orientee's competency on completion of orientation. Early anecdotal findings need not be included in the final evaluation if the orientee has demonstrated a sustained improvement. The written evaluation should be discussed by all involved with the orientee. There should be no surprises for the orientee in this session if communication has been open and consistent. The final evaluation can be an opportunity for all participants to reflect on the achievements and obstacles encountered during the orientation.

Addressing the situation of the orientee who has been unable to meet performance expectations is always stressful. Preceptors need the support of the nurse manager and the nurse educator when this occurs. Preceptors can feel guilty, frustrated, angry, disheartened, or experience a combination of all these emotions. In situations of this type, substantial effort is required by all involved with orientation. Although this can be exhausting, such outcomes are the exception rather than the rule; failure to address the situation carefully can have personal, professional, and organizational repercussions. Additional support may be sought from supervisory, administrative, and legal staff. Handling a poor performance situation should always be a team effort, with the orientee involved and informed on a regular basis.

If the orientee has been successful, this can be a time to enjoy the positive feedback and provide an opportunity for future planning. The orientee's success can predispose him/her to consider further educational pursuits, professional development activities, or involvement in unit projects. This is also an excellent opportunity to plant the seed for precepting in the orientee that may later develop into a willingness and desire to become a preceptor. One suggestion is to have orientees write personal descriptions of their orientation and their goals for the future and place these notes in sealed, self-addressed envelopes. These "letters," which can be mailed back to the orientees at a date specified in the future (i.e., 6 months, 1 year, on acceptance as a preceptor) are an excellent way to maintain a sensitivity to new staff members long after the feeling of newness has faded.

Evaluating the Preceptor

Like all staff members, the preceptor is evaluated at regular intervals, usually on an annual basis. Part of this annual performance evaluation should include a review of the nurse's willingness and ability to precept new staff members. If the job description includes precepting as an expectation, it should be reflected in the performance evaluation tool so there will be no surprises when the nurse is evaluated on precepting abilities.

The formal evaluation is important in validating the value and importance of the preceptor role, but it is not always timely in giving the preceptor the feedback that is needed immediately after orienting a new staff member. An evaluation process that parallels the orientee's evaluation process should be implemented. Throughout the orientation, the preceptor should be given feedback on his or her performance in the role. "On-the-go" meetings with the nurse manager and the nurse educator should include observations and suggestions on the preceptor's abilities, as well as the orientee's progress. At the end of each precepting experience, the preceptor should have the opportunity to discuss his or her precepting skills with the nurse educator and the nurse manager. The preceptor should be given an opportunity for self-assessment prior to receiving feedback. This will encourage and strengthen the preceptor's ability for self-evaluation and will give the preceptor insight into the process of self-evaluation in which the orientee participates.

The orientee's evaluation of orientation may include specific comments regarding the preceptor. These comments can be shared with the preceptor, but care should be taken to do this in a positive manner. Any unfavorable comments could cause the preceptor to become angry or hurt. The nurse educator should be able to relay the comments to the preceptor with an eye to improving future orientations, rather than blaming the preceptor for errors in the past.

SUMMARY

This chapter reviewed the design and implementation of a preceptorship program for nurse orientees in an acute health care facility. Before initiating a preceptor program, an assessment of the current needs and capabilities of the institution, the nursing department, and incumbent staff should be conducted. This will assure a preceptor program that is appropriate for the institution and congruent with its mission and goals.

Important components of a preceptor program include: criteria for preceptor selection, definition of preceptor responsibilities, program curriculum, orientation tools, and preceptor evaluation. To conduct an effective preceptor program, educational strategies that are consistent with the principles of adult education are essential. By adopting a preceptor model, the "initiation" of new nurses will be transformed into a positive and vital experience that will benefit both the orientee and the institution.

REFERENCES

Gardner, D. (1992). Conflict and retention of new graduate nurses. *Western Journal of Nursing Research, 14,* 76–85.

Knowles, M. S. (1970). *The modern practice of adult education.* New York: Association Press.

Kolb, D. A. (1993). *Learning style inventory user's guide.* Boston: McBer Training Resource Group.

Kramer, M. (1974). *Reality shock: Why nurses leave nursing.* St. Louis: Mosby.

Mulqueen, J. (1995). *Facilitating adults' adjustment to college: A manual for faculty.* Unpublished manuscript.

Myrick, F. (2002). Preceptorship and critical thinking in nursing education. *Journal of Nursing Education, 41*(4), 154–165.

Winter-Collins, A., & McDaniel, A. (2000). Sense of belonging and new graduate satisfaction. *Journal for Nurses in Staff Development, 16*(3), 103–111.

BIBLIOGRAPHY

Alspach, J. G. (2000). *From staff nurse to preceptor: A preceptor development program* (2nd ed.). Aliso Viejo, CA: American Association of Critical Care Nurses.

Beeman, R. Y. (2001). New partnerships between education and practice: Precepting junior nursing students in the acute care setting. *Journal of Nursing Education, 40*(3), 132–134.

Benner, P. (2001). *From novice to expert: Excellence and power in clinical practice.* Upper Saddle River, NJ: Prentice Hall.

Bolan, C. M. (2003). Developing a postbasic gerontology program for international learners: Considerations for the process. *The Journal of Continuing Education in Nursing, 34*(3), 177–183.

Brookfield, S. (1990). *Understanding and facilitating adult learning.* San Francisco: Jossey-Bass.

Delaney, C. (2003). Walking a fine line: Graduate nurses' transition experiences during orientation. *Journal of Nursing Education, 42*(10), 437–443.

Duff, M., & Kirsivali-Farmer, K. (1994). The challenge: Developing a preceptorship program in the midst of organizational change. *The Journal of Continuing Education, 25*(3), 115–119.

Greenberg, M., Colombraro, G., DeBlasio, J., Dolan, J., & Rich, E. (2001). Rewarding preceptors: A cost-effective model. *Nurse Educator, 26*(3), 114–116.

Haas, B. K., Deardorff, K. U., & Klotz, L. (2002). Creating a collaborative partnership between academia and service. *The Journal of Nursing Education*, *41*(12), 518–523.

Hrobsky, P. E., & Kersbergen, A. (2002). Preceptors' perceptions of clinical performance failure. *Journal of Nursing Education*, *41*(12), 550–553.

Merriam, S. (2001). *The new update on adult learning theory*. San Francisco: Jossey-Bass.

Wright, A. (2002). Precepting in 2002. *The Journal of Continuing Education in Nursing*, *33*(3), 138–141.

CHAPTER 5

A Model Preceptor Program in Home Care

Marilyn Hecker

This chapter explores the use of preceptorships for newly hired nurses in the specialty of home care. The desired outcome of the preceptorship is to improve the retention of new hires and to help facilitate their transition from neophyte to a contributing team member. Additionally, a well-developed preceptor program will create a milieu in which the orientees' self-esteem can be enhanced, contributing positively to their feeling of job satisfaction.

The purpose of this chapter is to

1. provide an overview of the specialty of home care,
2. describe a preceptor model used in home care,
3. define what is expected of the preceptee,
4. provide tools to measure the competence of the learner during and upon completion of the preceptorship, and
5. share anecdotal reactions from preceptors and preceptees about their personal experiences.

THE SPECIALTY OF HOME CARE

Overview

Home care provides a variety of health and social services delivered to patients who are acutely or chronically ill at home. These may include:

- nursing,
- assistance with activities of daily living (bathing, toileting) or instrumental activities of daily living (shopping, cleaning),
- therapy (physical, occupational, speech), and
- social services (entitlements, long-term planning).

These services are, in general, appropriately delivered in the home when the patient can safely remain there and when the skills necessary to deliver the care exceed those available from family and friends. As the nation's aging population grows and consumers elect to receive care at home, there will inevitably be increased demand for home health care providers.

The first home health agency was established in the late 1800s. By the year 2001 there were in excess of 20,000 providers servicing more than 7,000,000 patients in the United States. The enactment of Medicare in 1965 contributed to the industry's growth. Certified Home Health Agencies (CHHAs), which are able to bill Medicare for services, number slightly more than 7000 (National Association for Home Care, 2001).

Financial Considerations

With home care's expansion, costs skyrocketed. To contain this expenditure, Congress passed the Balanced Budget Act (BBA) of 1997. The BBA changed the way in which CHHAs were reimbursed for services and had an impact on the way agencies conducted business. This change has affected the body of knowledge necessary for new orientees to master, as well as the productivity requirements of staff.

New nurses entering home care must be able to function independently in the field (requiring finely tuned assessment skills), be knowledgeable in Medicare rules and regulations, understand reimbursement, and carry a demanding caseload. Though the rewards of home health care are great, expectations of the nurse are demanding. Staff turnover is a costly drain on a home health agency. The way in which the new hire is assimilated into the workforce is critically important to maintain job satisfaction.

Recruitment and Retention

The high cost of orienting new nurses and the extended period of time required before nurses reach the expected productivity level make each new hire a significant financial investment for a home care agency. Proper applicant screening is critical to minimize the number of inappropriate hires. The unique expectations of the role must be clearly communicated, especially to those applicants who do not have any home care experience. The historic belief that home care is a less demanding specialty than acute care misrepresents the role and, as such, is not appropriate for those who express interest in participating. Successful home care nurses are typically extremely well-organized, independent, and flexible. They enjoy autonomy, are capable of multitasking, are willing to make visits in varied neighborhoods with diverse home environments, and are willing to travel from place to place.

"It takes courage and confidence to provide patient care in an environment where there's no next shift to spot what was missed or physician reading your notes looking for significant symptoms" (Duckett, 2003, p. 500). Thoughtful interviewing and frank discussion are necessary hiring tools to identify those applicants who can be confident, organized, and flexible. Starting out with the right people is key to a successful home health nurse.

Providing a warm, supportive environment is not sufficient to keep new nurses from leaving home care during the orientation period. Conflict can exist between the nurse's perception of home care and the reality, similar to what was described by Marlene Kramer as "reality shock" (1974). Though Kramer was referring to the adjustment needed when going from academia to the workplace, similar stressors exist when transitioning from acute care to home health care. A well thought out approach to transition the nurse from new hire to team member with clearly defined expectations is essential for the new nurse to succeed. The use of preceptorships can provide the needed bridge.

Preceptor Selection

Selecting the correct person for the role of preceptor is central to the success of the entire program. The mere desire on the part of an accomplished staff member to become a preceptor is, in itself, insufficient. An effective preceptor is someone who is a knowledgeable home care professional, a good communicator, and patient, willing, and able to devote the necessary time to the learner.

The rhythm of a home care nurse's day will be changed by the presence of the learner. To make the expected visits per day and complete the requisite documentation while also meeting the needs of the preceptee is extremely challenging. Staff member productivity expectations should be realistically reduced when using an accomplished, experienced nurse as a preceptor, provided this is consistent with the culture and philosophy of the home care organization.

A possible alternate approach is to hire a full-time staff member who is a permanent preceptor to a continuous flow of new hires. This carefully selected and well-prepared individual can be assigned to a group of new hires from the completion of orientation to a point where the new nurse is ready to become a fully contributing member of the team. The length of time this may take can vary, depending on the skill set of the learner and the speed of the individual's progress. This approach allows time for one-on-one instruction, support, and case review because the preceptor is not stressed by his or her own caseload.

A disadvantage of this approach is that the preceptor is not actually a member of the home health care team and cannot help familiarize the learner with the culture and the social/interpersonal aspects of the job. However, this problem can be overcome if the preceptee attends staff meetings and has an opportunity to dialogue with the manager.

Informal discussions with preceptors frequently elicit their feelings of accomplishment in seeing the progress of the new nurse. As evidenced by the following quotes, preceptors grow and learn through the teaching process. "It is very gratifying to actually be able to do something that can have a positive impact on our profession." "I am very proud and fulfilled when I see a nurse succeed." "Kudos to preceptorships."

Preceptees express feelings of having been supported in their new role and nurtured while they gain the necessary knowledge for success in home care. The preceptorship can be a mutually beneficial experience for both the preceptor and preceptee.

A PRECEPTOR DEVELOPMENT PROGRAM

The curriculum for the preceptorship program illustrated here is designed to provide the preceptor with the skill set needed for a successful program. The department of staff development could administer this program. The content of the preceptor development program must provide instruction in adult learning theory, communication, and coaching strategies. Below is a sample curriculum (see Table 5.1).

PRECEPTORSHIP IN HOME CARE

Before the preceptor can begin the process of precepting the new nurse, orientees need to attend a number of training sessions facilitated by the department of staff development. This training is described below in Phase One: Initial Orientation. Phase Two

TABLE 5.1   Preceptor Development Program

---

1. "Remember When" Exercise: The purpose of this exercise is to have the preceptor designates identify and communicate their remembrances of their first few weeks at a new job so as to sensitize them to the feelings the preceptee will be experiencing.
2. Evolution of preceptorships in nursing: An historical perspective of preceptorships within the nursing profession is presented.
3. Definition of a preceptor: Preceptor is defined by explaining the differences among buddies, mentors, preceptors and teachers (see chapter 1).
4. Benefits of preceptorships: The benefits of preceptorships to both the preceptor and preceptee are discussed. An emphasis is placed on the mutual growth opportunities in these relationships as well as the satisfaction of championing the specialty of home care.
5. Adult learning principles: The principles of adult learning are reviewed and practical examples discussed (see chapter 2).
6. Reality shock in home care: Principles of Marlene Kramer's *Reality Shock* (1974) are applied to the "biculturalism" experienced when a new nurse's perceptions of home care meet up against the realities.
7. Communication strategies: Basic principles of good communication as well as productive ways to give feedback to the preceptee are reviewed.
8. "*A Five-step Micro Skills Model of Clinical Teaching*" (Neher, Gordon, Meyer, & Stevens, 1992) applied to home care nursing: This learning tool uses the five-step "micro skills" of clinical teaching described by J. O. Neher and associates for training physicians as a framework upon which good preceptor/preceptee conversations can be built.
9. Evaluation tools: Tools needed for appropriate evaluation of each preceptee are reviewed to ensure consistency in evaluation (see Table 5.2).
10. Job expectations/standards: The preceptee must be held to a reasonable workload. (see Table 5.3).

---

describes the point at which the preceptor has assumed his/her major responsibilities. Phase Three describes the orientee's transition to the staff position. In Phase Three, the preceptor remains in contact with the preceptee on an intermittent basis.

Phase One: Initial Orientation

The orientee should be provided with a strong foundation in clinical skills, home care principles, coordination of care, reimbursement, regulatory demands, and documentation requirements. This information can be presented in a variety of ways including:

- self study modules,
- group discussion,
- skills labs,
- lectures, and
- workshops.

Many required competencies can be successfully completed before making an actual visit to the patient's home. Orientation is most efficient when observation visits are interspersed among more didactic portions of the learning process. In this manner the learner can see principles acquired in the classroom immediately put to use in the field. A secondary benefit is that by placing an orientee in the field to observe a more experienced team member, informal sharing of the agency culture can be accomplished and networking among peers can begin.

This phase of orientation can last from 2–3 weeks or longer, depending upon the philosophy of the agency and the financial resources available. Special attention should be paid to the individual needs of the learner during this portion of the orientation. If a new hire comes to an agency with years of home care experience in a CHHA, then all classes in orientation may not be useful. This orientee should be placed in classes with similarly experienced learners, and the focus of classes should shift from general principles and requirements to policies and methodology specific to the individual CHHA. A multitract orientation should be considered where, for example, a class on cultural diversity would be heterogeneous (i.e., composed of experienced and inexperienced home care nurses) but a class on the Outcome and Assessment Information

Set (OASIS) would be more homogeneous in makeup. Use of technology to provide further individualization by self-guided study is also possible; however, the group process afforded the learner in the classroom setting has great value and should not be overlooked.

Phase Two: Preceptor/Preceptee Experiences

Upon completion of the more didactic portion of orientation the preceptee begins working with the preceptor. By the time this relationship is initiated, all the basic skill competencies have been completed in the laboratory. The orientee is ready to go into the field.

The preceptor selects an uncomplicated initial visit for the preceptee. On this visit, the field clearance is evaluated using the tool in Table 5.2. Upon successful completion of an initial visit, a wound care visit, and a home health aid supervisory visit made in the presence of the preceptor, the preceptee can then be cleared to do visits alone. The preceptor then continues to do ongoing case coordination with the preceptee and closely monitors the learner's caseload and progress. The tool in Table 5.3 is used as a benchmark against which to hold the preceptee accountable. This tool is helpful for the preceptor, who must evaluate the preceptee's progress, and is also useful for the preceptee, who must know exactly what is expected of him/her by the agency.

Phase Three: Transition to the Team

The preceptor/preceptee relationship continues until the learner has achieved a level of productivity and independence that warrants the preceptee being transferred onto the team. At this point, the new hire's supervisor becomes the primary resource and evaluator. Throughout the preceptorship, the preceptor should have been communicating the learner's strengths and weaknesses to the supervisor in order to facilitate continuity for the preceptee transfer to the team.

The first formal evaluation of the preceptee, which is the 90-day evaluation marking the end of the probationary employment period, is done by the preceptor and supervisor in tandem and signed by both.

TABLE 5.2 Field Evaluation Tool

Nurse: _____ Visit Type: _____

Date: _____ Evaluator: _____

Performance Rating Scale:

Yes: Consistently meets expectations. Performance of work activities and the manner in which they were achieved were at the level expected. This rating represents solid, competent performance.

No: Overall performance generally falls below the level expected. Needs some improvement to meet the standards for this job, either in the performance of work activities or the manner in which the work is performed. An improvement plan should be developed and follow-up counseling scheduled within three months.

N/A: Not assessed during the visit.

DIAGNOSIS: _____

PROCEDURE (s): _____

MEDICAL RECORD #: _____

	Yes	No	N/A	COMMENTS
Visit Preparation				
1. Contacts patient/significant other to confirm visit and time. Verifies the patient's address and communicates the purpose of the visit.	___	___	___	_____
2. Reviews case information, plan of care, physician's orders, reimbursement criteria.	___	___	___	_____
3. Corrects gaps in knowledge and information.	___	___	___	_____
4. Identifies purpose and focus of visit.	___	___	___	_____
5. Secures needed equipment and materials.	___	___	___	_____
6. Reviews the route to the patient's home.	___	___	___	_____

TABLE 5.2 *(continued)*

	Yes	No	N/A	COMMENTS
Visit				
1. Wears proper I.D. and introduces self.	____	____	____	_____
2. States purpose and focus of visit.	____	____	____	_____
3. Elicits main concern of patient/significant other.	____	____	____	_____
4. Places bag on a clean surface on a barrier and washes hands.	____	____	____	_____
5. Follows appropriate bag technique:				
Arranges necessary equipment on a barrier.	____	____	____	_____
Washes hands before bag reentry.	____	____	____	_____
Keeps bag zipped when not in use.	____	____	____	_____
Cleanses equipment before placing it back in bag.	____	____	____	_____
6. Systems Assessment				
Vital Signs	____	____	____	_____
Neurological	____	____	____	_____
Respiratory	____	____	____	_____
Cardiovascular	____	____	____	_____
GI/GU	____	____	____	_____
Skin	____	____	____	_____
Behavior	____	____	____	_____
Ambulation	____	____	____	_____
Pain	____	____	____	_____
Elicits specific and comprehensive data on identified problem areas.	____	____	____	_____

(continued)

TABLE 5.2 *(continued)*

	Yes	No	N/A	COMMENTS
7. ADL Status				
Hygiene Activities	_____	_____	_____	_____
Dressing Activities	_____	_____	_____	_____
Meal Prep, etc.	_____	_____	_____	_____
Assess for HHA/PCW	_____	_____	_____	_____
8. Psychosocial				
Family or significant other support.	_____	_____	_____	_____
Financial concerns/entitlements.	_____	_____	_____	_____
Assess for social work referral.	_____	_____	_____	_____
9. Nutrition/Hydration				
Appetite/Meal Routine	_____	_____	_____	_____
Weight	_____	_____	_____	_____
Rx/Diet/Fluids Teaching	_____	_____	_____	_____
10. Instruction				
Falls Prevention/Home Safety specific to patient dx.	_____	_____	_____	_____
Bill of Rights/Addendum	_____	_____	_____	_____
Patient Self-Determination Act	_____	_____	_____	_____
Admission Agreement	_____	_____	_____	_____
HHA BN	_____	_____	_____	_____
Notice of Noncoverage	_____	_____	_____	_____
OASIS Privacy Notice	_____	_____	_____	_____
Agency Name/Telephone	_____	_____	_____	_____
D.O.H. Complaint Telephone Number	_____	_____	_____	_____
Insurance Card/Carriers	_____	_____	_____	_____
Evening and Weekend Number	_____	_____	_____	_____
911	_____	_____	_____	_____
Physician	_____	_____	_____	_____
Signs/Symptoms of Disease Process	_____	_____	_____	_____
Complications of Disease Process	_____	_____	_____	_____

TABLE 5.2 *(continued)*

	Yes	No	N/A	COMMENTS
Procedures (specify)	___	___	___	_____
11. HHA/PCW Supervision				
P.O.C. initiated or revised to reflect current needs.	___	___	___	_____
P.O.C. reviewed with HHA/ PCW.	___	___	___	_____
HHA/PCW ID	___	___	___	_____
HHA/PCW Duty Sheets	___	___	___	_____
Other, specify:				
_____	___	___	___	_____
_____	___	___	___	_____
12. Medications				
Dose	___	___	___	_____
Frequency	___	___	___	_____
Route	___	___	___	_____
Effects—side effects	___	___	___	_____
Instructions	___	___	___	_____
13. Home Safety				
Mobility in home	___	___	___	_____
Physical layout of home	___	___	___	_____
Smoke detectors	___	___	___	_____
Instruct home safety	___	___	___	_____
14. Assessment of Assistive Equipment				
Canes: rubber tips, handgrip padding	___	___	___	_____
Walkers: rubber walker tips, wheels, handgrip padding	___	___	___	_____
Wheelchairs: braking system, seat belt arm/leg rest	___	___	___	_____
Commode: shower chair rubber tips	___	___	___	_____
Air/water mattress proper setting, leaking	___	___	___	_____
Seat cushions	___	___	___	_____
P.E.R.S. unit monitoring	___	___	___	_____

(continued)

TABLE 5.2 *(continued)*

	Yes	No	N/A	COMMENTS
Hospital Bed/Oxygen	___	___	___	_____
Instruct appropriate use of equipment	___	___	___	_____
Assess for therapy needs	___	___	___	_____
Patient outcome	___	___	___	_____
15. Evaluation of Teaching or Skill				
Assess patient's comprehension	___	___	___	_____
Verbal response to teaching	___	___	___	_____
Return demonstration	___	___	___	_____
POC Compliance	___	___	___	_____
Verbal review of procedure (if applicable)	___	___	___	_____
Need for Referral: YES NO	___	___	___	_____
16. Standard Precautions— Infection Control				
Thermometer cleansed w/alcohol after each use and uses thermometer cover.	___	___	___	_____
Diaphragm of stethoscope cleansed w/alcohol after use.	___	___	___	_____
Gloves changed after removal/disposal of old dressing.	___	___	___	_____
Hand washing between glove changes.	___	___	___	_____
Dispose of used dressing, gloves, bandages contaminated with blood or bloody fluids, urostomy pouches, BSD bags, by double bagging.	___	___	___	_____
Instruct infection control measures appropriately to POC	___	___	___	_____
17. Interdisciplinary Communication				
Communication with:				

TABLE 5.2 *(continued)*

	Yes	No	N/A	COMMENTS
Physician, coordinator, other disciplines	⎯⎯	⎯⎯	⎯⎯	⎯⎯⎯⎯⎯⎯
18. Documentation				
Reflects a skilled need.	⎯⎯	⎯⎯	⎯⎯	⎯⎯⎯⎯⎯⎯
Is accurate, legible and complete.	⎯⎯	⎯⎯	⎯⎯	⎯⎯⎯⎯⎯⎯
Timely Submission	⎯⎯	⎯⎯	⎯⎯	⎯⎯⎯⎯⎯⎯

Comments/Recommendations:

_____

_____

_____

_____

_____

_____

Signature of Administrator/DPS: _____ Date: _____

RN Supervisor Signature: _____ Date: _____

RN Signature: _____ Date: _____

*Note: Reprinted with permission from Metropolitan Jewish Health System. Brooklyn, New York.

Evaluation of the Preceptor

The essential functions of the preceptor are the parameters that should be used for evaluation. Although these functions are not all-inclusive, they are a basis upon which an evaluation tool can be developed. Major duties and responsibilities of the preceptor include:

1. observes field visits and reviews the required documentation,

2. monitors and develops new staff in the area of documentation for quality, justification for services, and reimbursement requirements in accordance with agency policy, and regulatory and accreditation standards,

3. assesses skills and abilities of new staff and provides additional education as needed, and

TABLE 5.3 Post-Orientation Expectations

Job Title: Coordinator of Care (COC)

After 4 weeks of employment the COC will be able to:

1. Demonstrate good infection control and proper bag technique in the field.
2. Maintain a productivity of 1–2 visits per day or 8–10 visits per week, (i.e., 2 initial visits).
3. Manage four (4) cases.
4. Assess the needs of the patient and develop a plan of care including assessing for Social Work, Physical Therapy, Occupational Therapy, and Home Health Aide.
5. Demonstrate the capability to submit for review Start Of Care (SOC) packets, 485s, and Outcome and Assessment Information Set (OASIS) within 24–48 hours of the initial visit.
6. Demonstrate good communication techniques with the patient and his/her significant others.
7. Demonstrate the ability to arrange for ancillary services.
8. Complete a weekly route sheet and revisit notes accurately and in a timely way.
9. Demonstrate good customer service.
10. Demonstrate good critical thinking skills.
11. Demonstrate emerging competency in implementation of the nursing process as it pertains to daily practice consistent with agency standards.
12. Demonstrate emerging computer skills.
13. Seek supervision as appropriate.
14. Demonstrate emerging knowledge of the Medicare and Medicaid regulations and their fiscal impact on the agency.
15. Demonstrate emerging knowledge of OASIS documentation and its clinical and fiscal implications.

After 12 weeks of employment the COC will be able to:

1. Maintain a productivity of 3–4 visits per day or 15–20 visits per week, (i.e., 3–4 initial visits).
2. Manage 12–15 cases.
3. Demonstrate competence in patient assessment.
4. Demonstrate progress in the ability to implement the nursing process as it pertains to daily practice consistent with agency standards.
5. Continue to consistently submit for review the SOC packets, 485s, and OASIS within 24–48 hours of initial visit.
6. Continue to refine documentation skills to meet the agency's standards.
7. Continue to demonstrate ability to complete a weekly route sheet and revisit notes accurately and in a timely way.
8. Demonstrate good time management skills.

TABLE 5.3 *(continued)*

---

9. Demonstrate emerging familiarity with the 60-day summary, recertification process, and follow-up assessment.

After 24 weeks of employment the COC will be able to:

1. Maintain a productivity of 5–6 visits per day or 25 visits per week, (i.e., 5–7 initial visits).
2. Manage 20–22 cases.
3. Uphold the agency's standards and demonstrate competence in all aspects of patient care, time management, and multidisciplinary conferencing/coordination.
4. Demonstrate the ability to complete a discharge summary and recertification.
5. Continue to demonstrate completion of weekly route sheets and revisit notes accurately and submit them in a timely way.
6. Continue to demonstrate good communication techniques with the patient, significant others, and other disciplines.
7. Continue to demonstrate good customer service.
8. Continue to demonstrate good critical thinking skills.
9. Demonstrate mastery of computer skills.
10. Demonstrate application of Medicare and Medicaid regulations.
11. Demonstrate mastery of OASIS documentation and its clinical and fiscal implications.

---

*Note: Reprinted with permission from Metropolitan Jewish Health System, Brooklyn, New York.

4. performs a review for all cases assigned to new staff to assess for appropriateness of the plan of care and remediates the preceptee as necessary.

SUMMARY

This chapter provides an overview of the specialty of home care and its unique challenges and rewards. The importance of careful selection of all new hires is discussed as well as the need to retain staff once they become productive team members. Preceptor selection is discussed and a preceptor development program is outlined. A tool for evaluation of the preceptees is provided and specific post-orientation expectations for the full-time home care nurse (Coordinator of Care) are described. The chapter provides an example of how to implement a preceptor program in home care and outlines a time frame for its completion.

REFERENCES

Duckett, K. K. (2003). Creating home health nurses—nature or nurture? *Home Healthcare Nurse, 21*(7), 500.

Kramer, M. (1974). *Reality shock: Why nurses leave nursing.* St. Louis: Mosby.

National Association for Home Care. (2001, November). *Basic statistics about home care.* Retrieved from www.nahc.org

Neher, J. O., Gordon, K. C., Meyer, B., & Stevens, N. (1992). A five-step "micro skills" model of clinical teaching. *Journal of the American Board of Family Practice, 5,* 419–424.

CHAPTER 6

A Model for Precepting in a Distance Nursing Education Program

Linda R. Conover

Providing learners with opportunities to apply new knowledge and skills is an important component when educating adults. This chapter provides an overview of the use of preceptors in a Master of Science in Nursing Distance Learning program that prepares nurses for roles as educators, leaders, and administrators, and parish nurses (nurses serving faith-based organizations). Although these roles are not usually associated with in-depth clinical learning experiences, providing students with opportunities to practice what they are learning (practica) under the guidance of an expert in the area is important.

PURPOSE

The purpose of this chapter is to

1. identify the components of a precepted educational experience;
2. discuss the phases of a well-designed precepted experience for distance learners;
3. discuss the responsibilities of learners, preceptors, and faculty members during precepted experiences in a distance learning program; and

4. discuss the key component of communication in a successful precepted learning experience with distance learners.

Description of the Precepted Practicum

The task of designing, planning, and implementing clinical experiences for learners is often a challenge for nurse educators. When students and their clinical learning experiences are at a distance from the home educational institution, the challenge may seem overwhelming. Once the issues are explored, however, the principles and practices associated with precepted experiences are no different for distance education than they are for an on-site program. The key element in any clinical experience involving the use of preceptors is communication. Similarly, effective communication among student, preceptor, and faculty member is key in a distance learning program. In addition, students must have a central role in the development and design of clinical experiences in their local areas.

Precepted practica in the Master of Science program are experiences that provide students with opportunities for expert guided learning and application of course content in settings away from the campus. These experiences are designed according to course descriptions. Learning objectives are developed by the student in collaboration with the faculty member assigned to the course. Expected outcomes for the practicum are also developed by the student in collaboration with the faculty member. Expected outcomes are different from learning objectives in that they specify what the final "product" will look like. For example, an expected outcome might be the development of policies and procedures. Learning objectives will address the knowledge the student hopes to gain about developing policies and procedures. These learning objectives and expected outcomes are shared with the designated preceptor who agrees to provide guidance to the student in meeting his/her learning objectives. The setting for the practicum depends upon the student's specialization, the course description, learning objectives, and availability of a qualified preceptor.

A preceptor is a professional nurse who, through education and experience, demonstrates expert knowledge in his or her field. The ideal preceptor enjoys working with students, is a positive role model, has effective communication skills, and holds a position at or above the level of expertise to which the student aspires. Ideally the preceptor also holds an appropriate graduate degree.

The student enrolled in a practicum must be an active learner. Individuality, self-expression, self-evaluation, and critical thinking are essential skills. Guidelines should be given to students to provide a roadmap for how to proceed. These guidelines should be grouped according to the following phases: preparation, approval and orientation, implementation, and evaluation.

Responsibilities of the Student Before the Practicum Experience

At least one month prior to the date the student intends to begin the practicum, he/she should enroll in the practicum course and contact the faculty member to discuss the learning experience. A course syllabus should be available that provides a general description of the intention of the course and basic learning objectives. The student should then develop personal practicum learning objectives, basic course objectives, and intended outcomes. This information, which is given to the faculty member, forms the basis for student–instructor discussion. Location of the intended experience and available potential preceptors are also discussed with respect to their meeting the criteria, as described in Table 6.1. The majority of

TABLE 6.1 Criteria for Preceptors in a Distance Learning Program

Education:	Master's Degree in Nursing preferred or BSN with Master's Degree in area related to practicum
Practice Level:	At or above the level for which the precepted experience is planned
Professional Attributes:	Role model, Positive attitude, Professional nursing image within the community and facility, Advocate for nursing and students, Excellent communication (oral and writing) skills, Ability to handle multiple tasks and decisions effectively and efficiently, Flexibility, and Perseverance to complete a project
Additional Areas:	Prior experience as preceptor or being precepted, Preceptor responsibilities fit work experience, and Willingness to work regularly with faculty member and student

communication between the student and the faculty member occurs via e-mail. Usually several drafts of learner objectives and intended outcomes are shared before they are clear and agreeable to both the student and the faculty member. Sometimes a phone "meeting" is necessary to achieve this clarity.

Once objectives and outcomes have been approved, the student makes contact with a potential preceptor. In cases where the student has not been able to identify a qualified preceptor, the faculty member assists the student to find potential local preceptors.

Once a preceptor has been identified, the student determines the preceptor's willingness to act in this capacity and shares the intended learning objectives and outcomes. The student then provides the potential preceptor with the required Preceptor Reference forms presented in Table 6.2, the Preceptor Application presented in Table 6.3, and an addressed, stamped envelope to return the information to the program office. Two references, the application form, and a current résumé are required to be submitted for preceptor approval.

When the preceptor has been approved and the contract described in Table 6.4 (from St. Joseph's College of Maine) has been signed, the faculty member notifies the student, who is then responsible for setting up the practicum orientation conference call. This conference call with the faculty member, student, and preceptor provides an opportunity to clarify the purpose of the practicum experience, the roles of each of the participants, the process, forms for documentation, and contact information for each participant.

Responsibilities of Students During the Practicum Experience

During the working phase of the experience, in addition to carrying out the intended learning activities, the student needs to maintain ongoing contact with both the preceptor and the faculty member. The frequency of contact with the preceptor varies depending upon the experience, the activities, and whether events occur that may require input from the preceptor to assist the student in achieving objectives. Contact with the faculty member occurs minimally every 2 weeks. In some instances more frequent contact may

TABLE 6.2 Preceptor Reference Form for a Distance Learning Program

Course Number _____

_____ has been asked to be a preceptor for one of our Master of Science in Nursing students. Your input will assist us in determining that this potential preceptor is appropriate for this student's practicum. Please rate the potential preceptor according to the criteria below and return this form in the envelope provided by the student. Thank you for your assistance.

Student's Name: _____

0 = don't know   1 = below average   2 = average   3 = above average   4 = outstanding

	0	1	2	3	4

1. Knowledge:
    Administration
    Education
    Parish Nursing					

2. Skill in applying theory in practice					
3. Role model/mentor					
4. Attitude about students					
5. Attitude about learning					
6. Professional nursing image					

7. Communication:
    Oral
    Written					

8. Ability to handle multiple tasks/ decisions easily					
9. Nursing advocate					
10. Follow through on projects					

Other Comments:

I have known the above named for _____ in the capacity of _____

_____   _____   _____
Signature   Print name   Credentials

_____   _____
Current position/title   Date

TABLE 6.3 Preceptor Application Form for Distance Learning Programs

Student's name: _____ Practicum Course # _____

Preceptor's name: _____

Preceptor's address: _____

Preceptor's telephone # _____ Preceptor's e-mail: _____

Preceptor's education: _____

Preceptor's practice level: _____

Preceptor's relationship to student: _____

Preceptor's professional attributes: _____

Has preceptor had previous experience as a preceptor? _____

Is preceptor willing to work regularly with faculty member and student? _____

Other comments: _____

Preceptor's signature: _____

Please return this form with two completed reference forms and a copy of your résumé to the Distance Nursing Education Office, attention to the faculty member who is responsible for the course.

be required depending upon the nature of the situation. For the most part, contact is through e-mail and submission of students' logs. For e-mail contacts, student, preceptor, and faculty member should be copied so that all benefit from the comments.

Students are required to keep a log of activities associated with appropriate learning objectives and outcomes. Students also should include a time count of practicum hours with each log submission. The minimum number of hours for a practicum is typically 135. Students are also required to meet any health and safety requirements of the setting in which they are located and must show that they hold a valid, unencumbered nursing license for the state in which their practicum occurs. Students in other

TABLE 6.4   Preceptor Contract

Student Name _____ Course Number _____

_____ and _____
Educational Institution   Health Facility

Agree to the responsibilities as identified below for students enrolled in the Department of Nursing, Master of Science program.

I   The College shall:
    A.   select educational prepared students for this practicum;
    B.   provide a nursing faculty member to collaborate with the preceptor at this facility;
    C.   initiate meetings with the student and the nurse preceptor to plan experiences, set goals, and integrate learning;
    D.   consult, assist, and problem solve with the student and preceptor during the practicum;
    E.   in collaboration with the preceptor and the student, determine if the student has successfully met the objectives and completed the outcomes for the practicum.

II   The Facility shall:
    A.   provide the student with access to the experiences necessary to meet his/her learning objectives;
    B.   foster a desirable learning environment by making agency resources available to the student, as permissible and appropriate;
    C.   provide an orientation for the student which includes policies and procedures;
    D.   not compensate or consider the student an employee during the hours the student is fulfilling his/her practicum requirements;
    E.   have the right, after consultation with Saint Joseph's College, to refuse to accept or continue any nursing student, who in the Facility's judgment is not participating satisfactorily or safely;
    F.   call to the attention of the faculty of Saint Joseph's College any problem reflecting on the qualifications of the student;
    G.   participate in the evaluation of the student's performance.

III   The Student shall:
    A.   identify his or her learning needs,
    B.   develop and maintain a working relationship with the preceptor,
    C.   maintain contact with the course faculty member,
    D.   meet health and safety requirements of the practicum facility,
    E.   function within the policies and procedures of the practicum facility.

IV   The parties of this agreement shall not discriminate against any student because of age, sex, race, religion, national or ethnic origin, or disability.

(continued)

TABLE 6.4 *(continued)*

V   By this agreement none of the parties incur any responsibility for financial exchange whether in monies or in kind.

VI   The College agrees to defend, hold harmless, and indemnify the Facility, its officers, employees, agents, and representatives against all liabilities, obligations, damages, claims, costs, and expenses (including reasonable attorney's fees) which result from or arise out of the College's performance of obligations under this Agreement or any College student's participation in the clinical training experience.

      The Facility agrees to defend, hold harmless, and indemnify the College, its officers, employees, agents, and representatives against all liabilities, obligations, damages, claims, costs, and expenses (including reasonable attorney's fees) which result from or arise out of the Facility's performance of obligations under this Agreement.

VII   This agreement shall be in effect beginning _____ and shall remain in effect for the duration of the student's practicum or until terminated by one or both of the parties who shall provide written notice of their decision.

This agreement may at any time be altered, changed, or amended by mutual agreement of the parties in writing.

IN WITNESS WHEREOF, this agreement has been signed by and on behalf of the parties identified above.

Date _____
For the Educational Institution: Faculty Member Dept. of Nursing

---

Date _____
For the Facility: Representative of the Facility

---

countries must demonstrate that they have met all requirements as defined by the country in which they are located.

Responsibilities of Students at the Completion of the Experience

At the completion of the practicum experience, the student collaborates with the faculty member and the preceptor to schedule a final conference call. At this time the student reviews all planned learning objectives and outcomes and discusses his/her progress. The preceptor is asked to comment on the degree to which the learning objectives and outcomes have been met. The faculty member asks for an overall opinion about the student's work and also asks for feedback on the entire process. The student is responsible for providing the Preceptor Evaluation of the Student Tool (Table 6.5) to the preceptor and for completing a Student Self-Evaluation Tool (Table 6.6). In addition, the student is responsible for ensuring that both the preceptor and the student self-evaluation tools are returned to the faculty member.

Responsibilities of the Faculty Member Before the Learning Experience Begins

The faculty member's responsibilities usually begin when the student enrolls in the course and makes contacts with his/her ideas about the practicum experience. This contact is often through e-mail and results in several communications to clarify the student's intentions. Learning objectives and planned outcomes are discussed and agreed upon. Often the student has a preceptor and location for the experience in mind. Sometimes the student needs assistance in locating an experience site and a qualified preceptor. Once the student has a site and potential preceptor, the faculty member waits to receive the Preceptor Application, a current résumé, and two completed Preceptor Reference forms. These materials are reviewed and the faculty member determines the appropriateness of the preceptor. When the preceptor has been accepted the student is notified by the faculty member and told to set up a conference call to start the experience. Students are instructed not to start working on the planned experience until this 3-way conference has occurred. During the conference call the instructor facilitates the discussion by urging the student to articulate his/her planned activities and outcomes. Any adjustments that need to be made based on input from all participants are agreed upon at this time. The faculty member also provides information to the student and the preceptor relative to expectations for frequency of contact, contact information for the faculty member, and any other clarifying information that the student or preceptor may need. At this time the faculty member explains that a three-way conference call may be requested at any time. The need for such

TABLE 6.5 Preceptor Evaluation of the Student

Directions: Using the following rating system, please rate the student at the completion of the Practicum Project (PP) in the areas listed below by placing an "X" in the grid for the course objectives and program outcomes.

Section 1

The student demonstrates:

1. Minimal knowledge, language, and skill related to the PP. Requires continuous oversight and direction from the preceptor.
2. Basic understanding of the knowledge, language, and skill required for the PP. Requires frequent direction by the preceptor.
3. Knowledge, language, and skill to complete the PP with minimal direction from the preceptor.
4. A high level of knowledge, language and skill for independent completion of the PP in collaboration with the preceptor.

Course Objectives	1	2	3	4
1. Assessed a population for health-related needs				
2. Applied population-focused care principles in a clinical setting				
3. Participated in collaborative problem-solving approach to providing care				
4. Achieved desired outcomes				
5. Achieved individualized objectives				

Please feel free to add any other comments here and/or on the back of the page.

(continued)

TABLE 6.5 *(continued)*

Section II

Program Outcomes	Fully Achieved	Partially Achieved*	Minimally Achieved*	Not Achieved*	Not Applicable
1. Improve health care delivery and patient outcomes					
2. Engage in ethically based professional behaviors					
3. Use critical thinking to apply advanced nursing knowledge in practice/education settings					
4. Demonstrate professional nurse behaviors of caring, respect, integrity, and positive regard for others					

*Note: Please qualify any responses that were not fully achieved.

Student's signature _____ Date _____

Preceptor's signature _____ Date _____

conference calls occurs rarely and usually results from changing circumstances at experience sites necessitating a change in the student's plans.

Responsibilities of the Faculty Member During the Experience

During the practicum the faculty member's responsibilities are primarily focused on fostering communication with the student and preceptor to discuss student progress and any potential or

TABLE 6.6 Student Self-Evaluation Form

Directions: Using the following rating system, please rate yourself at the completion of the Practicum Project (PP) in the areas listed below by placing an "X" in the grid for both the course objectives and your individualized outcomes.

Rating System

The student demonstrates:

1. Minimal knowledge, language, and skill related to the PP. Requires continuous oversight and direction from the preceptor.
2. Basic understanding of the knowledge, language, and skill required for the PP. Requires frequent direction from the preceptor.
3. Knowledge, language, and skill to complete the PP with minimal direction from the preceptor.
4. A high level of knowledge, language, and skill for independent completion of the PP in collaboration with the preceptor.

Rating

Course Objectives	1	2	3	4
1. Assessed a population for health-related needs				
2. Applied population-focused care principles in a clinical setting				
3. Participated in collaborative problem-solving approach to providing care				
4. Achieved desired outcomes				
5. Achieved individualized objectives				

TABLE 6.6   *(continued)*

Please rate your progress on the following Program Outcomes	Fully Achieved	Partially Achieved*	Minimally Achieved*	Not Achieved*	Not Applicable
1. Improve health care delivery and patient outcomes					
2. Engage in ethically based professional behaviors					
3. Use critical thinking to apply advanced nursing knowledge in practice/education settings					
4. Demonstrate professional nurse behaviors of caring, respect, integrity, and positive regard for others					

*Note: Please qualify any responses that were not fully achieved.

Student's signature: _____ Date _____

actual problems. Sometimes the faculty member may be asked to assist when problems arise. Frequently, however, the student and the preceptor have already developed a solution for problems that have arisen before checking with the faculty member. In most instances, the solutions and adaptations suggested by students and preceptors will turn out to be the most appropriate. As the student and the preceptor are the closest to the problem, they usually have the best information for solving it. During this problem solving, the preceptor's role modeling of adapting to change and processing this with the student usually results in an excellent learning experience.

Responsibilities of the Faculty Member Upon Completion of the Experience

Throughout the entire process students are progressing in meeting their learning objectives and accruing the required hours. Students send biweekly updates in their logs, including the number of hours completed. In most cases the hours and the completion of the learning objectives and outcomes coincide. On occasion the faculty member may have to question continuation of the project based on the number of student hours completed. This is rare and usually happens when there has been an adjustment to the plan midway through the experience. In some cases students complete planned activities even though it necessitates extending their hours beyond the requirement. Most students want to finish their projects and feel a sense of responsibility to the people with whom they have been working.

A final conference call with student, preceptor, and faculty member is conducted for the purpose of reviewing the experience and evaluating student performance and progress. The faculty member again facilitates this discussion with the student and the preceptor. One of the most important aspects of this final phase is to thank the preceptor for his/her time and effort with the student.

Once written evaluations have been received, the faculty member posts a grade for the practicum. She/he also initiates a thank-you communication to the preceptor from the director of the program, as the entire process would not work without the commitment of the preceptor.

Responsibilities of the Preceptor Before the Experience

Once agreeing to be a preceptor for a student, the preceptor completes the Preceptor Application form and submits it along with a current résumé and two references. The forms are provided by the student, who should include an addressed, stamped envelope. Once the preceptor has been approved, he/she should be in contact with the student to review planned learning activities and outcomes. When agreement is reached on those items, the preceptor participates in the first conference call with the student and the faculty member. At this time the preceptor has an opportunity to voice any concerns and to identify any potential barriers to the planned activities. Planned activities are adjusted as necessary.

Responsibilities of the Preceptor During the Learning Experience

Working with the student during the experience requires the greatest amount of effort on the part of the preceptor as the student proceeds to work on planned objectives and outcomes. Ongoing contact with the student occurs frequently (i.e., once or more daily) or less frequently (i.e., weekly) depending upon the setting, student abilities, and planned experiences. The preceptor is asked to keep a log of contacts with the student to verify that contact is being made on a regular basis.

Responsibilities of the Preceptor at the Completion of the Learning Experience

When everyone agrees that learning objectives and outcomes have been met, the preceptor participates in the final conference call with the faculty member and student. The preceptor is also asked to complete an evaluation of the student's intended learning, which is returned with his/her log to the instructor. The preceptor is free to suggest a final grade for the student but the faculty member is the one who determines the course grade.

SUMMARY

This chapter has presented the process for developing and implementing a distance learning preceptorship for graduate students. The roles and responsibilities of the student, preceptor, and faculty were presented. Ongoing, clear communication and clearly defined objectives and outcomes were identified as important contributing factors to the success of this type of program. Advantages to this model of precepting included flexibility for the learner in selecting the practicum experience and exposure to professional contacts all over the globe.

REFERENCES

Cafferella, R. S. (2002). *Planning programs for adult learners: A practical guide for educators, trainers, and staff developers* (2nd ed.). New York: Wiley.
Knowles, M. (1980). *The modern practice of adult education*. Chicago: Follett.

CHAPTER 7

Beyond Preceptorships

Anne E. Belcher

There is a wide variety of educational/orientation programs available to new graduate nurses, as well as to experienced nurses in practice. These programs include but are not limited to internships, externships, fellowships, and apprenticeships. In addition, mentorship offers unique opportunities for continuing professional development to both mentor and protégé. The general purposes of these programs are (a) to bridge the gap between academic preparation and initial clinical practice while easing role transition; (b) to improve the recruitment, retention, and job satisfaction of nurses in health care agencies; and (c) to produce a positive cost–benefit ratio in the recruitment/orientation/retention budget.

Each type of program has entrance/selection requirements, a curriculum, clinical experiences, and evaluation strategies. Agencies that offer one or more of these programs report that these programs positively impact the participants' professional behaviors; values, attitudes, and beliefs about health care and nursing; job satisfaction; and participation in continuing education. The objectives of this chapter are to describe these programs, to generate questions for research about such programs, and to describe mentorship.

INTERNSHIPS

Nursing internships, which were first developed and implemented in the early 1960s, are viewed as extended orientation programs intended to bridge the gap between the role of the student and that of the competent nurse (Schempp & Rompre, 1986). Internships were initially created for medical-surgical and specialty areas. The programs varied in length from 8 weeks to 1 year. Class-to clinical hours ratios also varied (Kotecki, 1992). Reflecting the popularity and numbers of these programs throughout the '60s, '70s, and '80s, the National League for Nursing (1983) published *Internships for the New Nurse Graduate*, which listed hospital nursing internships available throughout the United States. This document is currently out of print.

An internship program is defined as a semi-structured, supervised orientation that includes didactic and clinical components (Ross, 1986). Sams, Baxter, and Palmer-Smith (1990) indicate that a professional internship should be based on the principle that all nurses must have at least entry-level competency in their specialty before assuming full staff nurse function. They recommend the use of an adult learning approach, which includes identification of clinical competencies and interaction with preceptors.

The goals of nurse internships are to build consistent decision-making skills, to promote adaptation to the work environment, and to support the development of competent and proficient practitioners (Kopp et al., 1993). Many hospitals have implemented nurse internships in an effort to improve recruitment and retention of nursing staff based on the belief that they improve job satisfaction, lessen feelings of powerlessness, and decrease turnover rates. The use of concepts basic to professional nursing practice is deemed to be cost effective as well. Sams and colleagues (1990) determined that such a model "(1) provides administration with a means of defining entry-level practice according to national standards; (2) provides the manager with a validation mechanism that the nurse is able to practice all aspects of nursing, not just accomplish specific tasks; (3) provides the preceptors with a clear guide for directing clinical experiences; and (4) illustrates a specific set of professional criteria that enables nurses to collaborate with preceptors and to validate their abilities daily" (p. 94).

Ressler, Kruger, and Herb (1991) described a Critical Care Internship Program whose goals were: "to provide new graduate nurses with the opportunity to increase knowledge and acquire critical care nursing skills, to provide graduate nurses with a practical clinical experience under the supervision of an experienced nurse, and to increase the number of educated critical care nurses available for employment" (p. 177). Classes presented included basic principles of critical care nursing and a focus on how the principles could be applied to the clinical setting. The preceptor played a pivotal role in validating assessment skills, reinforcing application of knowledge at the bedside, and serving as a role model. Process and outcome evaluation strategies indicated that the Critical Care Internship Program provided the new graduate nurse with the knowledge and clinical experience needed to provide care for critically ill patients.

Craver and Sullivan (1985) found that new graduate nurses who participated in an internship program had fewer absences from work and a lower attrition rate than those new graduates who were not interns. However, no differences were found in job performance evaluations, job satisfaction, or nursing skills. Kopp and colleagues (1993) evaluated a Critical Care Nurse Internship Program (CCNIP) that provides didactic instruction and supervised clinical experience to graduate nurses seeking staff nurse positions. They determined that the CCNIP promoted competency and assisted in the recruitment and retention of staff nurses in critical care. Rosenthal and Connors (1989) discovered that a collaborative Pediatric Intensive Care Unit/Neonatal Intensive Care Unit (PICU/NICU) internship was a successful strategy for meeting the ongoing challenge of integrating the new graduate nurse into the critical care environment in a supportive and educationally sound manner. Cooney (1992) described a successful orientation program for new graduate nurses desiring work in obstetrics. The use of a Skills Checklist; class days for didactic presentation of special topics; and an Orientation Evaluation Scale that measures the new employees' level of supervision needed, organization, precision, and understanding produced nurses who were prepared to meet professional standards of care, who were retained longer than in the past, and who valued ongoing participation in staff development.

Beth Israel Hospital in Boston developed a Clinical Entry Nurse Residency Program for new graduate nurses in the mid-1990s. This standardized, 2-year, planned first work experience provided graduates of baccalaureate or higher degree programs with the necessary skills and behaviors needed for fulfilling the professional nursing role. The program included hands-on clinical teaching, ongoing mentorship, and career planning. The resident worked with a clinical nurse sponsor, whose focus was on the process of "socialization" into professional nursing and individual career development.

The objectives of the residency were to:

1. demonstrate the centrality of caring in professional nurse/patient/family relationships;
2. demonstrate competence in providing quality, cost-effective nursing care;
3. demonstrate leadership skills in all aspects of professional practice;
4. formulate a plan for continued development and overall career goals; and
5. appreciate the larger context of the health care delivery system.

Learning methods included assigned readings, shadowing experiences, reading and writing clinical exemplars, presenting patients at rounds, reviewing research articles, attending committee meeting and lectures, and meeting with various resources in the institution (Duprat, 1994).

Internship programs are an excellent opportunity for collaboration between nursing service and nursing education (Hartshorn, 1992). The program could be developed with school and hospital educators sharing responsibility for clinical and classroom experiences. Graduates' participation in the program might enable them to earn academic credit. Hospital-based educators benefit by working with school of nursing faculty who have an in-depth understanding of the new graduate. School of nursing faculty benefit by working with hospital-based educators who are up-to-date regarding changes in the clinical setting.

Kotecki (1992) completed an extensive review of the literature regarding internships since their inception in the 1960s and reached the following conclusion: "Many of the (internship) programs are creative and innovative but, when compared with regular orientation programs, do not show significant differences in clinical ability, role transition, or recruitment. However, a relationship does seem to exist between internship programs and retention of graduate nurse employees" (p. 205).

NURSING EXTERNSHIPS

In general, an externship is a period of time during which a student works under the direction of someone with experience in the profession. A variety of terms have been used to describe such a structured work experience: internship, externship, work experience, fieldwork, practicum, directed projects, and cooperative education. All have the common purpose of providing structured student experiences outside of the classroom (Konsky, 1976). According to Cottrell and Wagner (1990), it is in the externship that students learn to apply what they have learned to a real life situation; it "provides a type of culminating experience to the education process" (p. 30). The benefits of an externship are as follows:

1. students attain the confidence and experience needed to handle an entry level position in the profession successfully,
2. successful student externs may have an advantage in the job market over those who choose not to complete an externship, and
3. professional contacts and networking opportunities can be invaluable to the extern when seeking an initial or future professional position.

The sponsoring educational institution gains personal contact with practicing professionals, which is important for public relations, for future student placement, and for opportunities to conduct applied field research. The externship site also benefits from student externs serving as additional staff to accomplish daily tasks and to initiate projects that may have been placed on the back burner due to inadequate employee time. Externs also offer fresh ideas and new insights to the sponsoring agency and its employees.

Constraints or problems presented by externships include such specific issues as inadequate supervision of the extern as well as such comprehensive issues as lack of research on the development, administration, and effects of such a program on the extern and on the agency. Cottrell and Wagner (1990) raised some interesting questions regarding externship programs that are applicable to nursing:

*   Are site visits made during the externship and, if so, who makes the visits?

- Can students receive salary and/or living expenses?
- Do formal procedures exist for the approval/certification of externship sites prior to student placement?
- What criteria are used in selecting externship sites?

Nursing externships have been offered by schools of nursing and health care agencies for many years. Most of these programs employ students in summers only and were designed to supplement nursing staff in the agency during those months when vacation coverage was needed. Nurse externs work for a salary that is usually equivalent to or somewhat higher than that of other nonlicensed personnel. Some hospitals provide special classes for the externs and use a preceptor model for clinical supervision. The employing agency anticipates that the externs will apply for a full-time position after they have completed their nursing education. In this time of a nursing shortage that is projected to last for many years, agencies may find the externship program increasingly cost-effective because of externs' shortened orientation and enhanced retention.

FELLOWSHIPS/APPRENTICESHIPS

Fellowships and apprenticeships are types of internships in which a professional gains practical experience under the direction of another professional. Fellowships and apprenticeships come, according to Buckalew (1984), "in all shapes and sizes—paid, unpaid—formal, informal—long, or short term" (p. 28). The fellow or apprentice agrees to work on a particular project for an organization, such as doing research or collecting data, and in turn gains valuable knowledge and experience while working with experts in the specific field. Buckalew has the following suggestions for a nurse who is interested in pursing a fellowship or an apprenticeship:

- Have the name of an individual to contact or direct the inquiry to the personnel department.
- Identify your interest and background in the health care system, not limiting your qualifications and experiences to nursing.
- Be prepared with a concise and updated résumé, stress research completed or in which you have participated, and list all publications.

Smaller councils within governmental agencies work on specific projects that may be of particular interest to the nurse applicant; these fellowships or apprenticeships are usually unpaid, and have small staffs and limited work space. However, they can be advantageous to the applicant if he/she has flexible work hours and can use the experience for college credit or to help further a cause, for example, women's health, aging, or world hunger.

Examples of agencies that offer fellowships/apprenticeships that may be available to interested and qualified nurses include:

- American Association of Retired Persons
- American Hospital Association
- American Nurses Association, including the Minority Fellowship Program
- Congressional Placement Office
- Department of Health and Human Services
- National Academy of Sciences
- White House Fellowships

State legislators and other nursing organizations may offer additional fellowships and apprenticeships. The focus of those listed above is on involvement in the political arena. As noted by Buckalew (1984): "Getting involved means work over and above the usual. It may demand sacrifice of time or money, in some cases both. However, the long-term benefits to the nursing profession will be worth it" (p. 29).

RESEARCH QUESTIONS

Each of the programs described above offers opportunities for research that to date has been only descriptive or lacking entirely. Research questions could and should be generated to address a variety of issues, such as the following:

- How should applicants be selected for these programs? What criteria should be used?
- How can articulation with schools of nursing be used to enhance new graduates' preparation for and faculty participation in these programs?

- What differences in curriculum design, content, and experiences are needed to assure the expected outcomes of such programs? How is the optimal length of such programs determined?
- What is the cost-effectiveness of these programs? How is it measured? How are costs and benefits weighed to determine the value of the program?
- How do these programs affect recruitment and retention of staff? How is job satisfaction measured?
- How are preceptors best selected? How are they prepared, evaluated, and rewarded for their participation in these programs? How are they matched with potential interns?

More attention should be directed to the evaluation process. Many programs use subjective evaluation measures that make it difficult to assess the actual benefit of the programs.

- What clinical performance evaluation tool is valid and reliable for determining nurses' success in these programs?
- How can preceptor, nurse manager, and nurse/other health care professional colleague involvement and satisfaction with program participants be determined?

MENTORSHIPS

Mentorship is a highly complex and developmentally important relationship that may include but is not limited to (a) teaching specific skills; (b) developing a protégé's intellectual capabilities; (c) intervening to assist in the protégé's entry into and advancement within the organization; (d) providing advice, encouragement, and constructive criticism; (e) introducing the protégé to organizational operations, politics, and key players; and (f) serving as an exemplar who models the values and professionalism that the protégé can emulate. According to Bowen (1985), mentoring

occurs when a senior person (the mentor) in terms of age and experience undertakes to provide information, advice, and emotional support for a junior person (the protégé) in a relationship lasting over an extended period of time and marked by substantial commitment by both parties. If the opportunity presents itself, the mentor also uses both formal and informal means of influence to further the career of the protégé. (p. 31)

Yoder (1990) differentiates the concept of mentoring from those of role modeling, sponsorship, precepting, and peer strategizing. Role modeling does not require a personal relationship between the model and the imitator. The model's role is a passive one, based on the assumption that the imitator will identify with the model and adopt the model's behaviors and values. Sponsorship has all of the characteristics of mentorship with the added aspect of finding the "right spot" for the protégé in the organization. Precepting has been previously defined in this book. As Fawcett (2002) notes: mentors are not only responsible for "showing a new nurse how to perform a task," but also for "explaining why the task is performed and modeling the behavior" (p. 952). Peer strategizing usually consists of two persons who are peers in age and experience who engage in a reciprocal or mutual relationship. This "trading of information" sustains the relationship over time.

The four stages of the mentor–protégé relationship are as follows:

Stage 1: Solicitation: This first stage involves the process of determining whether there is "good chemistry" between the mentor and protégé. During this time, the mentor is probing with the protégé around the thoughts and ideas they are both bringing to the relationship.

Stage 2: Inquiry: During this second stage, the mentor's primary function is to clarify expectations and define goals with the protégé. This stage is often characterized by some anxiety with the mentor and the feeling of being unable to meet expectations and goals.

Stage 3: Informational: This stage involves the protégé's knowledge and skill development: learning the ropes, gaining insight into the broader organizational experience, understanding the organizational game plan, and becoming familiar with who wields the power.

Stage 4: Conversion: The fourth stage is symbolized by the protégé's autonomy and independence. The protégé, through the achievement of personal goals, begins to separate from the mentor. This stage may be characterized by disillusionment with the relationship, a simple parting of the ways, or a new and redefined relationship (Yoder, 1990).

Potential dilemmas and barriers of the mentor–protégé relationship were identified by May, Meleis, and Winstead-Fry (1982) as (a) independence versus protectiveness, in which the mentor may overprotect the protégé, thus stifling innovative ideas; (b) collegiality versus exploitation, in which the assertive and competitive protégé may cause the mentor to be too cooperative or the overly competitive mentor uses the protégé as a pawn to reach self-serving goals; (c) mentorship versus educator role, which are distinctly different; and (d) individuation versus protégé status, in that mentors must encourage protégés to be autonomous, not clones of themselves.

Darling (1984) categorizes mentors in such a way that each nurse can identify personal preferences and style with regard to this role. The four mentor types she identifies are:

1. *the traditional mentor:* a person who is sufficiently experienced in a career to be able to give wise counsel to the protégé;

2. *the step-ahead mentor:* an older person either in age or experience, one who can "pave the way," protect, or give valuable guidance to the younger person starting on the same path;

3. *the comentor:* a peer in age and experience who is engaged in a reciprocal or mutual relationship with the other person; the two either take turns providing guidance and assistance as it is needed or provide help to each other in specific areas;

4. *the spouse mentor:* a special form of comentor, which can be very significant in marriages, being either unilateral or reciprocal.

The type of mentor one tends to use is related to the stage of one's career life cycle.

Fawcett (2002) asserts that effective mentors have the following characteristics: patience, enthusiasm, knowledge, a sense of humor, and the ability to engender respect. Outstanding mentors also learn about their protégé's personal background, competencies, and professional ambitions.

DeMarco (1993) notes that the classic mentor/protégé relationship has emerged in various health care settings based on the need for nurse recruitment and retention and continues to "take the shape and form of the older, more experienced person guiding, supporting and nurturing a younger, less experienced one" (p. 1243).

With regard to reciprocity, the antecedents are the following:

1. At least two people are interacting in an exchange that has meaning for both (thoughts, feelings, behaviors).
2. Interfering factors outside of the exchange must be less potent than the meaning of the exchange.
3. The skill to facilitate reciprocity rests on the decrease of interfering factors.
4. Participation in the relationship proceeds from a philosophic premise that human existence encompasses multiple and personal meanings, shared participation, multiple outcomes amenable to change, mutual learning, and intuitive, rational, and empirical characteristics (p. 1244).

The four consequences of a mentor/protégé relationship should be

1. shared meanings through mutual understanding,
2. two individuals sharing control and responsibility for the outcomes of the relationship,
3. trust that is developed and sustained, and
4. an empowerment to cope. (DeMarco, p. 1244)

With regard to empowerment, Hawks (1991) acknowledges the attributes of interpersonal process and the antecedents (power skills), trust, knowledge, respect, and self-confidence. Solidarity comes with group identification of common goals and needs.

The value of mentorship in nursing is its positive impact on professionalism, reduced turnover, and increased job satisfaction. The challenge facing the new graduate nurse is to find a senior/ experienced person or persons who will serve as guides through his or her career. As noted by Vance (2000), mentor connections play a role in leadership succession in the nursing profession, as well as contributing to nurses' success and satisfaction throughout their career paths.

SUMMARY

As nursing shortages accelerate in the years ahead, more emphasis will be placed on programs that support new graduates as well as experienced nurses, with a focus on recruitment and retention. Those programs described in this chapter provide a history and framework for new endeavors in this area. Mentorship will always be an important aspect of the profession of nursing and its value should be instilled in each nursing student, faculty member, and nurse in practice.

REFERENCES

Bowen, D. (1985). Were men meant to mentor women? *Training and Development Journal, 39*(1), 30–34.

Buckalew, J. (1984). Internships for nurses. *Home Healthcare Nurse, 2*(4), 28–29.

Cooney, A. T. (1992). An orientation program for new graduate nurses: The basis of staff development and retention. *The Journal of Continuing Education in Nursing, 23*(5), 216–219.

Cottrell, R. R., & Wagner, D. I. (1990). Internships in community health education/promotion professional preparation programs. *Health Education, 21*(1), 30–33.

Craver, D. M., & Sullivan, P. P. (1985). Investigation of an internship program. *The Journal of Continuing Education in Nursing, 16*(4), 114–118.

Darling, L. A. (1984). Mentor types and life cycles. *The Journal of Nursing Administration, 14*(11), 43–44.

DeMarco, R. (1993). Mentorship: A feminist critique of current research. *Journal of Advanced Nursing, 18,* 1242–1250.

Duprat, L. (1994). The clinical entry nurse residency program. Offering bright futures for new graduate nurses. *Report on Professional Nursing at Boston's Beth Israel Hospital, 12*(2), 1–3.

Fawcett, D. L. (2002). Mentoring—what it is and how to make it work. *AORN Journal, 75*(5), 950–954.

Hartshorn, J. C. (1992). Characteristics of critical care nursing internship programs. *Journal of Nursing Staff Development, 8*(5), 218–223.

Hawks, S. H. (1991). Powers: A concept analysis. *Journal of Advanced Nursing, 16,* 754–764.

Konsky, C. (1976). Practical guide to development and administration of an internship program: Issues, procedures, forms. *ERIC,* #ED 249 539, 1–30.

Kopp, M. E. A., Schell, K. A., Laskowski-Jones, L., & Morelli, P. K. (1993). Critical care internships: In theory and practice. *Critical Care Nurse, 12*(8), 115–118.

Kotecki, C. N. (1992). Nursing internships: Taking a second look. *The Journal of Continuing Education in Nursing, 23*(5), 201–205.

May, K. M., Meleis, A. I., & Winstead-Fry, P. (1982). Mentorship for scholarliness: Opportunities and dilemmas. *Nursing Outlook, 30*(1), 22–28.

Ressler, K. A., Kruger, N. R., & Herb, T. A. (1991). Evaluating a critical care internship program. *Dimensions of Critical Care Nursing, 10*(3), 176–184.

Rosenthal, C. H., & Connors, C. (1989). Pediatric/neonatal graduate nurse internship: A collaborative effort. *Pediatric Nursing, 15*(2), 194–196.

Ross, V. (1986). An internship for leadership in nursing. *Nursing Outlook, 14*(2), 40–42.

Sams, L., Baxter, K., & Palmer-Smith, P. (1990). A competency-based model for nurse internships. *Journal of Nursing Staff Development, 6*(2), 93–94.

Schempp, C., & Rompre, R. (1986). Transition programs for new graduates: How effective are they? *Journal of Nursing Staff Development, 2*, 150–156.

Vance, C. (2000). Discovering the riches in mentor connections. *Reflections on Nursing Leadership*, Third quarter, 24–25.

Yoder, L. (1990). Mentoring: A concept analysis. *Nursing Administration Quarterly, 15*(1), 9–19.

Index

Springer Publishing Company

Evaluation and Testing in Nursing Education

2nd Edition

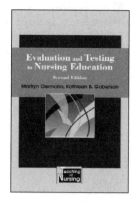

Marilyn H. Oermann, PhD, RN, FAAN
Kathleen B. Gaberson, PhD, RN, CNOR

"This comprehensive textbook and reference presents the information in a clear, well-organized, concise manner...the authors have created a book that will be of tremendous help to those seeking assistance."
— Doody's Health Sciences Book Review Journal
praise for the 1st Edition

This award-winning book for both novice and experienced nurse educators has been thoroughly updated in its second edition. The only book in nursing education that focuses entirely on the key areas of evaluation and testing, this text explains how to prepare all types of test items and explores how to assemble, administer, and analyze tests, measurement concepts, grading, and clinical evaluations.

Educators will learn the basics of how to plan for classroom testing, write all types of test items, evaluate critical thinking, written assignments, and clinical performance, and more. New content in this edition includes:

- Writing alternate item formats similar to the NCLEX® Examinations
- Developing tests that prepare students for licensure and certification exams
- Strategies for evaluating different cognitive levels of learning
- Evaluating written assignments and sample scoring rubrics
- Up-to-date information on testing in distance education environments with a special focus on internet and on-line based testing

Teaching of Nursing
August 2005   432pp   0-8261-9951-8   hardcover

11 West 42nd Street, New York, NY 10036-8002 • Fax: 212-941-7842
Order Toll-Free: 877-687-7476 • Order On-line: www.springerpub.com